This work by José Argüelles provides the first
thorough, scholarly study of the unique personality and extraordinary achievement of
Charles Henry (1859-1926). Seeking a comm
ground for all sensory experience, Henry formulated a "scientific aesthetic" based on the
biomathematics of the sense organs. That doctrine is psychophysics, through which Henry
saw beyond the dualism which had thrown
science and art into separate camps.

Mr. Argüelles's presentation of Henry's
aesthetic provides a new and original perspective on neo-impressionism and its aftermath.
Among those influenced by Henry's ideas,
especially those concerning the perception of
color, were Georges Seurat and Paul Signac
as well as some of the pioneer abstractionists—
Robert Delauney, Frank Kupka, and Albert
Gleizes. The study also casts new light on the
poet Jules Laforgue (one of Henry's closest
friends) and on the symbolism of the 1880s
and 1890s.

As Mr. Argüelles shows, Henry was equally
at home with the leading poets, painters, and
scientists of Paris in the 1880s. Extraordinarily
erudite, Henry's multidisciplinary lectures
on aesthetics fascinated Seurat, Signac, Pissarro,
and others. As Paul Valéry wrote, Henry
"distinguished the only doctrine which could
at the same time permit a correspondence
(Continued on back flap)

Charles Henry
and the Formation
of a Psychophysical
Aesthetic

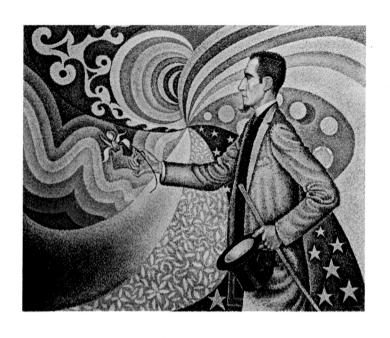

Paul Signac's *Against the Enamel of a Background Rhythmic with Beats and Angles, Tones and Colors. Portrait of M. Félix Fénéon in 1890, Opus 217.*
Private collection, New York
Photograph by Charles Uht

Charles Henry and the formation of a Psychophysical Aesthetic

José A. Argüelles

The
University
of Chicago
Press
Chicago
and
London

The University of Chicago Press, Chicago 60637
The University of Chicago Press, Ltd., London
© 1972 by The University of Chicago
All rights reserved. Published 1972
Printed in the United States of America

International Standard Book Number: 0–226–02757–0
Library of Congress Catalog Card Number: 72–189026

Contents

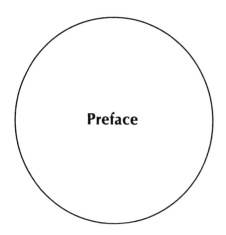

Preface

MANY are the attempts that are made and the words that are spoken with regard to the age-old ideal of harmony: the union of all faculties, of all senses, of all men, and of all knowledge. The highest dreamers would proclaim that true art and science are One. Whatever the time or the situation, if the science or the craft or the technique employed be utilized to bring about in all respects a harmonious resolution of tensions and polarities, then it will qualify as an aspect of what the alchemists once called the Great Work, the one art and science of harmony.

The seekers of harmony have taken many different forms and have practiced many different arts and techniques, depending upon the time and the situation. Often it is surprising to discover that what at first might have seemed a rather curious or even anomalous work contains within it yet another articulation of the science and art of harmony. Such is the revelation contained within the works of Charles Henry (1859–1926), who reformulates the doctrine of harmonic unity as psychophysics and the doctrine of harmonic work as the psychophysical aesthetic. Thus when both the physical properties and psychic functions of that which reaches our senses—light, color, form, and sound—are understood in their mutual interdependence, the creation of harmonic

Preface

works becomes possible. This is the essence of the reformulation of the doctrine of harmony that is contained in the
various works of Henry: *L'Esthétique scientifique, Rapporteur
esthétique, Cercle chromatique,* "Le lumière, la couleur, la
forme," to mention a few.

That all of this was apparent to at least some of Henry's
contemporaries is evident; yet the full impact of his reformulation of the doctrine of harmony was never fully assessed,
particularly in its aesthetic ramifications. Indeed, when first
encountering the works of Henry, I was ill-prepared for what
I was to discover: a fully elaborated philosophy relating man
to the cosmic whole. It took me several years to realize that
Henry's "scientific aesthetic" was not necessarily an adaptation of empirical scientific principles to the domain of art,
but something of a reformulation of science as well. When
finally—thanks to a chance perusal of Mirabaud's, *Charles
Henry et l'idéalisme scientifique*—I glimpsed that Henry's
science was a marriage of Pythagoras and Descartes, I eagerly
conceived the notion of this book, and it is my hope that the
reader will be able to glimpse through the uniqueness of
Henry's method a philosophy as old and revered as that of
the sages of ancient times.

The first version of this work was submitted as my doctoral dissertation to the University of Chicago, where it was
accepted in 1969. I am most indebted to Professor John
Rewald under whose guidance I first came across Henry,
while studying the art of the neo-impressionists in 1964–65,
and without whose inspiration and example this work should
not have seen the light of day. I am equally indebted to
Professor Joshua C. Taylor, whose encouragement and help,
especially in the more general aesthetic and philosophical
problems, was of inestimable value. I must also express gratitude to the Samuel H. Kress Foundation whose grant in
1965–66 enabled me to study firsthand in Paris many of the
documents of the symbolist period. I am also indebted to
discussions with Dr. Robert Sommer, Chairman of the Psy-

Preface

chology Department, University of California at Davis, and Dr. Charles T. Tart of the same department, who have been most helpful in elucidating for me the state of psychological research as it has developed in recent times.

Above all, I must acknowledge eternal gratitude to my wife, Miriam, whose help, thoughts, criticisms, and inspired enthusiasm make this as much her work as mine.

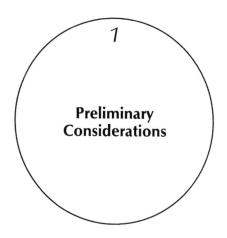

1

Preliminary Considerations

I N the history of human thought there are many attempts to define the limits of possible knowledge. But there are no interesting attempts to conceive what the extensions of these limits would mean and where it would necessarily lead."[1] In the conviction that the aesthetic doctrine of Charles Henry is one of these "interesting attempts," I intend to present and elucidate, where I can, the essentials of this doctrine. Aspects of this aesthetic formulation have been examined and applied to the works of Georges Seurat, most notably by William Homer (*La Parade, Le Chahut, La Cirque*)[2]

1. P. D. Ouspensky, *A New Model of the Universe* (New York, 1943) p. 15. Like Henry, Ouspensky was a mathematician concerned with the creation of a new unitive vision of things in which science and mysticism are combined; also like Henry, Ouspensky was interested in alternative theories of evolution, since the Darwinian model seemed totally inadequate. And finally, there must be recognized in Henry's work a conscious attempt at extending the given state of human knowledge and at indicating where this extension might lead.

2. William Homer, *Seurat and the Science of Painting* (Cambridge, Mass., 1964). Homer's book is the most exhaustive analysis of Seurat's aesthetic. More than any other modern writer, he attempts to relate the ideas of Henry to those of Seurat (see pp. 188–249), though by self-admission Homer's treatment of Henry's ideas is by no means thorough; the whole topic tends to be confused and even vague. Thus Homer states: "Yet many of the similarities between Seurat's esthetic and Henry's theories still must be regarded as coincidental, rather than the result of direct influence of

Chapter One

and Dorra (*La Cirque*).³ The relevance of this aesthetic has also been noted with respect to the neo-impressionist movement in general, primarily by Rewald⁴ and Herbert.⁵ On the other hand, the basic tenets of Henry's doctrine have never been clearly stated or examined, due in large part to the fact that Henry's role has never been well defined. In attempting to present the aesthetic ideas of Henry, I have found it necessary to understand his motivations and, hence, his role as well. However, I shall engage in historical analysis and interpretation only insofar as it serves to clarify my one purpose: the exposition of Henry's aesthetic doctrine. I shall avoid as much as possible that analysis which implies reinterpretation. Also, except in the case of the *Portrait of Fénéon* by Signac, I shall not indulge in any lengthy and involved application of Henry's aesthetic ideas; primarily because this has already

the scientist on the artist" (p. 199). Homer tends to give more credit with regard to "influence" on Seurat to books that Seurat could have read—Helmholtz, Sutter, Blanc, Chevreul—than to the living influence of a man like Henry, Seurat's contemporary and peer. Though there is really little evidence to prove either contention, I am of the opinion that Henry was of inestimably greater influence on Seurat than were the writings of a man like Charles Blanc, for instance, simply because living intercourse and experience are almost always more vital than what is gained from books.

3. Henri Dorra and John Rewald, *Seurat: L'oeuvre peint: biographie et catalogue critique* (Paris, 1959), pp. c–cvi. Both Dorra and William Homer agree that *La Cirque* is an example of an almost strict application of Henry's theories of the correspondence of direction and color.

4. John Rewald, *Post-impressionism. From Van Gogh to Gauguin* (New York, 1956).

5. Robert L. Herbert, *Neo-Impressionism* (New York, 1968), pp. 21–23. Herbert discusses Henry's ideas under the topic "The Abstract Components of Art." Although it is evident, neither Herbert nor Homer realize that the "abstract" values of Henry's theories are really not abstract but *symbolic*, thus quite the opposite of abstract the way the word is defined by Herbert: "devoid of reference to the real world." Nor do Homer and Herbert realize that Henry's ideas are as transcendental as they are "scientific." On this matter see Gustave Kahn, "Au temps de Pointillisme," *Mercure de France* 171 (1924):5–23, and Kahn, "Réponse des symbolistes," *L'Evénément* 28 (September, 1886). Kahn, of course, relates Henry directly to a transcendental aesthetic. Sven Lövgren, *Genesis of Modernism* (Uppsala, 1959), follows Kahn's interpretation of Henry.

2

Preliminary Considerations

been done by Homer and Dorra, with whose conclusions I am generally in agreement, and, too, because only in the Fénéon portrait is there what seems to be a case of very *conscious* application of the aesthetic doctrine in question. It is this element of self-consciousness which separates the Fénéon portrait from kindred works by Seurat, Signac, and others.

Because in many ways Henry and the aesthetic he develops are unusual, a good deal of time will be spent on Henry's early life and education and also on the sources of his ideas. Since none of this has ever been well explored—neither Henry's life nor the psychophysical ideas of the nineteenth century as they apply to art and culture—I believe such matters, however general, are of the greatest importance in presenting this material. On the other hand, there are a host of general questions raised by the inherent nature of the material that pertain not only to art but to science and the general nature of knowledge as well. These questions are significant for purposes of historical reevaluation and contemporary relevance; to have shirked them would have been a disservice to my goal.

The presentation of "historical" material is not a laboratory matter, the dissection of certain data and their consequent classification. On the contrary, what is involved is the satisfaction of a certain need or necessity. The historical material answers a present and immediate need, and cannot be separated from the present and immediate perceptual process which engages it. Why has Henry not been studied previously? Because previously there was no need for the conclusions which Henry's ideas occasion. The model or paradigm which Henry's doctrine exemplifies has not been the model or paradigm in common use, therefore it has not been necessary to employ it or one like it.[6] But certainly that does

6. I have found most useful Thomas S. Kuhn, *The Structure of Scientific Revolutions* (Chicago, 1970). Kuhn's thesis is that "normal science" presupposes a conceptual framework or paradigm which obviously and in-

Chapter One

not make Henry's model any less true or useful; all one can say is that it simply has not satisfied the common collective prejudice of recent times, though in the 80s and 90s it did. It is well to keep in mind the idea of a poet-friend of Henry's, Paul Valéry: "*The image of this world* is part of a family of images, an infinite group, all the elements of which we possess—but unconsciously—consciousness of possession is the secret of the inventors."[7]

Now obviously in the presentation of Henry's aesthetic doctrine, the author is acutely aware of his position and role vis-à-vis Henry. Like Valéry and, most certainly, Henry, I have come "to suspect all accustomed reality of being only one solution amongst many others of universal problems."[8] It is in the interest of this idea that I bring to public attention the solution posed by Henry.

Since there is no biography of Charles Henry, so to speak,[9]

---

evitably provokes a crisis and a revolution in purpose and method. It is my contention that psychophysics is that new model which provokes a crisis to the "normal science" dating from the time of Descartes. I also agree with Kuhn that "normal science" discredits the new and defends itself to the end, as it were. The merit of Kuhn's book is that it places science within a context of historical psychology where it becomes evident that so-called scientific truths are often just as arbitrarily founded as any other popular prejudice.

7. From the "Introduction to the Method of Leonardo da Vinci," in *Selected Writings of Paul Valéry* (New York, 1950), p. 90 (first published in the *Nouvelle revue*, 1895). This particular writing of Valéry's contains many "echoes" of Henry's own work, especially in the following passage: "The gods have received from the human mind the gift of the power to create, because that mind, *being cyclical and abstract*, may aggrandize what it has imagined to such a point that it is no longer capable of imagining it"; then follows a discussion on the cyclical and curvilinear aspect of ornament. If anyone could be considered a philosopher of cycles it must be Henry, with whose work Valéry was most certainly familiar. See also, Paul Valéry, "Charles Henry, in "Hommage à Henry," *Cahiers de l'étoile* no. 13 (January–February, 1930):20–24. Valéry states that he met with Henry but once, yet the impression made upon him was profound because of the magnitude of Henry's endeavor.

8. Valéry, "Introduction to the Method of Leonardo da Vinci," p. 90.

9. My biographical information is taken, unless otherwise noted, from the special *Cahiers de l'étoile* issue (see above, note 7). For further information, see the Bibliography.

4

Preliminary Considerations

let me state a few facts which comprise the official biography of our subject. He was born May 16, 1859, in Bollweiler, Alsace-Lorraine. Next to nothing is known of his early life other than that he was brought up in moderate circumstances and that as a young man, blue-eyed and blond-haired, he looked more like his mother than his father. Henry was in Paris in 1875 pursuing a free course of study, first under the famed experimental physiologist and doctor, Claude Bernard, and then under a less-known figure, Paul Bert, who was also apparently an experimental scientist. In addition to science, Henry seems to have studied languages—Greek, Latin, Sanskrit, and German—at this time, and it also appears that his father willingly consented to support young Henry even though the son's course of study was not a specific one. The year 1878 marks the beginning of Henry's erudite publications. Also about this time Henry began to make literary acquaintances, most notably Jules Laforgue, Henry's neighbor on the rue Berthollet; he also came to know Gustave Kahn, as well as the mysterious Mlle. Mullezer, Sanda Mahali. Henry was "le savant" of the "club des hydropaths," that curious protosymbolist group. In 1881 Henry was named a sublibrarian at the Sorbonne.

From the 1880s into the middle 1890s Henry was a most active participant in his times; indeed, he was something of a symbolist figure, his friendships and acquaintances extending to such persons as Félix Fénéon (with whom Henry helped found *La vogue* in 1886), Seurat, Signac, and Paul Valéry. During this time many of Henry's articles appeared in the leading avant-garde journals such as the *Revue indépendante* and the *Revue blanche*. In 1892, Henry was named "Maître de conférences a l'école des hautes études" at the Sorbonne. In addition to his publications on aesthetics, mathematics and psychology, he was engaged in chemical research which resulted in the discovery of a phosphorescent sulphur of zinc, as well as several other industrial products such as varnishes and the like. Also Henry's interest turned more to the study

5

of blackbodies, radiation, and various electromagnetic and chemical phenomena. From 1895 to the time Henry received his doctorate in 1910, his life is more obscure and seems to be marked by less activity than in the 80s and early 90s; perhaps it was a necessary period of gathering and reflection— and of riding the bicycle, a sport which with Henry was a passion. Henry's doctoral thesis was in two parts, *Sensation et énergie* and *Mémoire et habitude*. At this time too, a position was made for him: Director of the Laboratory of the Physiology of Sensations at the Sorbonne. From this time to his death, Henry was engaged in synthesizing his various endeavors, the culminating work being the *Essai de généralisation de la théorie du rayonnement* [Generalization of the theory of radiation], published in 1924.

As late as 1922 Henry contributed an article on light, color, and form to the journal *L'esprit nouveau,* but generally speaking the period of Henry's aesthetic experimentation belongs "au temps du symbolisme," and because of this it is this earlier and better known period of his life to which I shall be devoting my attention. This is not to slight the latter part of Henry's career; quite the contrary. In many ways the latter half of Henry's life is most fascinating and carries with it a dream of a different kind than that which marks the first part of the life of this "historical riddle." In fact, in the last years of his life, official pressure seems to have forced Henry to set up his laboratory at Coyes near Versailles where he could work without harassment; it is here in November of 1926 that Henry died, or, to use his own words, underwent another "physiochemical change."

A problematic life, to say the least, and to grasp as a whole a most difficult task. Though I have labored to do justice to but one aspect of Henry's career, I have always worked under the growing knowledge and conviction that whatever I said or did could only be in the nature of a preliminary sketch.

This aside, the immediate concern will be Henry's aesthetic ideas and system. But since for Henry, aesthetics is only an

Preliminary Considerations

aspect of a larger system, growing of necessity from the developmental exigencies of that system, a perspective on the larger system must be developed. This is so because finally for Henry aesthetics is the seeking out and implementation of those rhythms which will enhance life and expand consciousness. From this point of view, aesthetics is a necessary psychobiological function which furthers the evolution of the organism, and it must be understood that for Henry the working out of this concept of aesthetics (and its consequent implications for whatever art would develop from it) was but a necessary step in the working out of an entire cosmological conception. In its promulgation of the idea that the science of art is a psychobiological physics, Henry's aesthetic has been classified variously as Darwinian interpretation[10] and most certainly as an example of nineteenth-century aesthetics turning to science for support, confirmation, or reevaluation.

However, as my research progressed I realized, slowly but surely, the complexity of the problem. As I have already indicated, to give a man like Henry his full due is to raise a host of questions concerning some of the basic paradigms or models of our intellectual, historical, and scientific structures. Primarily, Henry was able to combine in himself what is generally considered the scientific attitude with the mystic one, a fact which in itself tends to confront some of our basic ideas. Yet in viewing the sum of Henry's work one is struck by the logical consistency of the development of this work and its aim. Precisely because of the inner logic which is a chief characteristic of Henry's work from beginning to end it may be assumed that at an early age he had a presentiment, even a revelation of an idea, however summarily revealed, which acted as a guiding force through the various endeavors of his life.

10. See Horace M. Kallen, *Art and Freedom* (New York, 1942), 2:580–581; also Peyton E. Richter, *Perspectives in Aesthetics, Plato to Camus* (New York, 1967), p. 278.

Chapter One

One of the biographers of Jules Laforgue, perhaps Henry's closest friend in the years which we shall be considering, speaks of the "religious crisis" the poet was undergoing in the earliest years of his friendship with Henry;[11] Gustave Kahn writes that, in this same period, Laforgue was an "adept of modern Buddhism."[12] This was in the years 1879–80. At this same time Kahn says of Henry, that "he was visited often by a man who knew all the languages and had become a vice-consul in the Orient, an intermittent and excellent translator of difficult texts of the Persian poets."[13] And, too, there are Henry's writings at this time, particularly those dealing with the history of certain mathematical notations which indicate that he was quite aware of any number of ancient and/or oriental mathematical systems as far afield as Tibet and Chaldea, with whose astronomical concepts Henry also seems acquainted. From these few hints we may glean that when Henry was scarcely twenty years of age the seed was already planted. It is significant that in his final work of summing up, the mathematically abstruse *Théorie du rayonnement,* Henry concludes that all his efforts in psychomathematics were but the planting "of some solid stakes in a land whose existence is generally denied or suspect, and which is hinted at only by Buddhist wisdom and by a few seekers."[14] That he was aware of this "land" from the first is certain, but it was not specifically in the footsteps of the Buddha that Henry achieved his work, but in those of Pythagoras—not that the footsteps lead to different places; quite the contrary.

11. François Ruchon, *Jules Laforgue, sa vie—sa oeuvre* (Geneva, 1924), pp. 24–25. This and all other translations from the French in the text are my own, unless otherwise noted.
12. Gustave Kahn, *Symbolistes et décadents* (Paris, 1902), p. 182.
13. Ibid., p. 25.
14. Charles Henry, *Essai de généralisation de la théorie du rayonnement* (Paris, 1924), p. 139. With regard to this matter of the relation of psychophysics and Buddhism, the reader's attention is drawn to Lama Govinda, *The Psychological Attitude of Early Buddhist Philosophy* (London, 1961), in which the system as well as the language by which the system is propounded is definitely psychophysical.

Preliminary Considerations

"*All* is number. Number is in all. Number is in the individual. Ecstasy is a number."[15] Such are the words of the poet Baudelaire whom Henry so greatly respected. This concept of number may be taken as the base of Henry's "neo-Pythagorean" science, echoed also in the words of Leibnitz, to whom Henry refers. "Musica est exercitum arithemeticae occultae nescentis se numerare animi."[16] Henry pursues a mystically mathematical mode of investigation, as he makes clear towards the conclusion of the *Cercle chromatique*. In this work, Henry speaks of an "indefinitely evolutive law"[17] whose origin he attributes to Pythagoras. Indeed, Henry's mathematical formulation of the law of evolution which, incidentally, bears no necessary relationship to that expounded by Darwin and Spencer, is based on the same Pythagorean principle of the Tetracys of the Decad, that is, on the representation of the number ten, a primary whole number, by ten dots arranged in a pyramid.[18] Henry states that "one can construct the curve of evolution according to time, if one notes that, after my fundamental theorem, purely successive groups are symbolized by the sums of successive primary numbers. After this law, each time that one of the sums will be able to be placed in the form of a product, it will tend to be realized

15. Charles Baudelaire, *Intimate Journals,* trans. C. Isherwood (Boston, 1957), p. 3.
16. Quoted in J. Hericourt, "Une théorie mathématique de l'expression: le contraste, le rythme et la mesure, d'après les travaux de Charles Henry," *Revue scientifique* 44 (1889):593. Hericourt's is one of the few articles which discourses at length and most favorably on Henry's ideas. Also quoted in idem, "Henry, le contraste, le rythme et la mesure," *Revue philosophique* 28 (1889):375.
17. Charles Henry, *Cercle chromatique de Charles Henry, présentant tous les compléments et toutes les harmonies de couleurs . . .* (Paris, 1888), p. 163.
18. Henry's utilization of Pythagoras is most unique. In a sense, Henry's own mathematics with its emphasis on whole numbers and their succession is an intermediary between Pythagoras and quantum mechanics, which also formulates energy transformations in terms of the succession of whole numbers. For Pythagoras, see Eduard Zeller, *Outlines of the History of Greek Philosophy* (New York, 1955), pp. 51–53.

under that form."[19] Without getting too far ahead, let it suffice to say that Henry's approach is most singular, and to get at it requires a great deal of clearing away.

Returning to the central topic of this study, let it simply be said that one of Charles Henry's contributions was in the realm of art and aesthetics. As a result of his aesthetic work, he was able to formulate the concept that the way in which art can best serve the evolution of consciousness is by becoming a medium expressive of joy, completely integrated with the rhythms of life. In Henry's words, art has a dynamogeneous function, and the function of dynamogeneous movement or action is to expand consciousness. Thus art based on dynamogeny becomes a mechanism of evolutionary furtherance. Henry, who was an evolutionist in the fullest sense of the word, that is, one participating in the continual transformation of phenomena/experience with the intention of expanding consciousness, was naturally impelled to work out a concept of art and aesthetics dynamically flexible and concordant with the principle of a universal and all-pervasive evolutionary event. By "transformation" is meant the ongoing states of integration, disintegration, and reintegration or synthesis which constitute the dynamic process of evolution, or, to speak more organically, growth. It can also be stated that Henry held the view that evolution is not merely the "survival of the fittest," and that it is not a purely random event. Because of this, he can hardly be called a Darwinian.

On the contrary, Henry synthesizes two traditions or ideas in order to arrive at his "indefinitely evolutive" law in which aesthetics plays such an instrumental role. The first tradition is that of the classical mathematicians—Pythagoras, Anaximander, and the other Greeks; the Arabs; Kepler, Descartes, and Leibnitz. The second tradition is that of "classical" scientific experimentation, more precisely, the nineteenth-century science of psychophysics—"the science which considers

19. Henry, *Cercle chromatique*, p. 164; we will pursue Henry's mathematics further in chapter 3 below.

Preliminary Considerations

the relation of body and mind"[20] or, to put it another way, which studies the transformation of phenomena into states of consciousness or vice versa. In comparison to the accepted evolutionary paradigm, Henry's idea of evolution is one that is more organically ordered, in a mathematical as well as biological sense, and consequently it is one that recognizes as its goal the expansion of consciousness. This emphasis on consciousness rather than on morphogenetic differentiation is due to the psychophysical approach which is finally as deviant a departure from classical Western science and thought as was produced in the nineteenth century. Like the Buddhist, the psychophysicist "does not inquire into the essence of matter, but only into the essence of the sense-perceptions which create in us the representation of the idea of matter."[21]

But what is psychophysics? And how does it relate to art? This requires some necessary statements about the assumptions and implications of the little-regarded phenomenon of nineteenth-century psychophysics, the investigation of which in turn touches upon basic assumptions of Western thought and art. To explain the role of Henry, who is in many ways the archetypal psychophysicist, I shall proceed first with a brief general exposition on the role and function of psychophysics and then go into a more extensive study of Henry and the aesthetic ideas which he formulated.

20. In the first chapter of Gustav Fechner, *Elements of Psychophysics* (New York, 1966), vol. 1. I shall have occasion to discuss this matter in greater detail in the next chapter.

21. Govinda, *Early Buddhist Philosophy*, p. 133. From a larger point of view, the historical movement of psychophysics in the West in the nineteenth and twentieth centuries signals a large-scale and conscious *rapprochement* with the basic tenets of Oriental thought. There is a complementary movement from the Orient, as exemplified in the work of Ramakrishna, Vivekananda, and the modern Yoga movement begun under the auspices of Sri Aurobindo which stresses the psychophysical nature of Yoga and consciousness. See Vivekananda, *The Yogas and other Works* (New York, 1953); Sri Aurobindo, *Life Divine* (New York, 1949); Akit Mookerjee, *Tantra Art: Its Philosophy and Physics* (New Delhi, 1966).

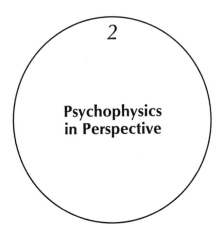

2

**Psychophysics
in Perspective**

SINCE there is no broad evaluative study of the nine-teenth-century science of psychophysics, one must be indicated, however briefly and tentatively. As I have already suggested, psychophysics, though utilizing the classical scientific method in order to study the nature of sense experience, does so, at least originally and by its very assumptions, to provide a way out from the heavy materialistic orientation which had become such a basic feature of nineteenth-century European thought and culture. I should also state that my own method is a broadly psychological one; for this method the specific nature of things, ideas, systems, and fashions is a direct function of the state of consciousness which produces such phenomena at a given time in a given place. This method is universally applicable, and classical Western science is no exception; it, too, is the necessary creation and function of a specific mode of consciousness, and is subject to the limitations of that state of consciousness.

Quite simply, knowledge is a function of the system which creates it. The nature and variability of that knowledge corresponds to the extensibility of the system (and the state of consciousness of which the system is a function) which finds that knowledge necessary for its own functioning. What is not within the system is not considered to be known, know-

Psychophysics in Perspective

able, or necessary. The scientific method is such a system, though it is generally held to be an absolute cornerstone of our civilization. Briefly, this method entails the hypothesis of an observer/experimenter; the experiment, which is the manipulation of raw data in a closed "laboratory" situation; and the results. If the results conform to the hypothesis, there is a quantum of new "verifiable" knowledge; if results do not conform to the hypothesis, a new one is formulated.

The blind spot of systems is their methodology; the blind spot of classical science is the scientific method. This method splits the universe into two absolutes: the subject and the object, the knower and the known. What is "knowable" is external phenomena and the laws pertaining to such phenomena. Within the limits it set for itself, Western science was incredibly successful. As it progressed through the eighteenth and into the nineteenth centuries, it built up, or so it is thought, a great body of outer, objective knowledge (to use its terminology), leaving the inner—"subjective"—area of the "mind" and the emotions relatively unknown and, in a sense, unknowable.[1]

In line with this development, modern Western psychology has generally followed the route of the objective approach, leaving out of its consideration, almost entirely, the subjective domain of the mind. One contemporary psychologist, Gardner Murphy, pinpoints this phenomenon by stating that modern psychology is based upon "physicalist models." Murphy sums up this situation as it has developed in the twentieth century:

> The physicalist models were at first almost purely negative. Bekhterev in the Russia of 1907 and John B. Watson in the United States of 1912 banished con-

1. See T. Roszak, "The Myth of Objective Consciousness," in *Making of a Counter-Culture,* New York, 1969, pp. 203–38. Although behavioralism arose as the statistical formulation of emotional patterns, this is still essentially only dealing with what is objectively observable, that is, behavior, and not with the nature of emotions themselves.

13

sciousness as an object of study and undertook to write an objective or behavioralist psychology. Of course, they used physicalist models, physical-chemical definitions of life processes, and physiological research methods. They were in a sense, "throwing into the wastebasket" all the nonphysicalist concepts which they could not understand. . . . Though some of them adopted a systematic philosophy, either materialist or neo-realist, many of them were content simply with this banishing process by which the traditional problems of mind, self and awareness were turned back to the philosopher, and found a simple straight path by which the young biologically-oriented scientists of the day were to achieve their status among their scientific brothers.[2]

The situation is obviously a complex one, and though he is most astute in his awareness of the problem, Murphy does not take into account the idealist strain of nineteenth-century psychophysics prior to the rise of behavioralism. Yet his reflections are significant, and the truth is that modern thought and research is still dominated to a large extent by the purely objectivist approach.

Naturally, there must be reaction of a slow yet revolutionary and synthesizing nature. Where and how to pinpoint this reaction is another matter, for by its nature it is a collective and ongoing phenomenon. However, within this context it can be stated that one of the turning points is the introduction of the idea or science of psychophysics in the middle of the nineteenth century, for in its broadest sense psychophysics was a profound reaction to the scientific approach of the day.

2. Gardner Murphy, "Human Psychology in the Context of the New Knowledge," *Main Currents in Modern Thought* 21 (March–April, 1965): 76. This is a most illuminating statement relating to the whole issue of scientific consciousness and the possibility of expanding beyond its present state.

Psychophysics in Perspective

Gustav Fechner published his *Elements of Psychophysics* in 1860,[3] a year after Darwin's *Origin of Species*. Fechner's basic idea is very simple: the magnitude of the stimulus is proportional to the magnitude of the sensation and is something that can be mathematically determined. There is nothing unusual or disturbing in this. However, Fechner also applies his method to the notion of measurement: the unit of measure is conditioned by ultimate degrees of sensitivity; sensitivity ultimately depends upon the measurer's own subjective experience. Objective knowledge, therefore, is dependent upon subjective experience. What, then, is the

3. Published as *Elemente der Psychophysik* (Leipzig, 1860), in two volumes, the first dealing with Outer Psychophysics and the second with Inner Psychophysics. The English translation published in 1966 (see above, chapter 1, n. 20) is of the Outer Psychophysics, and bears an introduction by E. C. Boring, who states that "Fechner's *Elemente der Psychophysik* of 1860 stands at the head of the new science of psychology." The translator's foreword by Helmut E. Adler underlines the ambiguous respect in which Fechner's name is generally held. Though coining the word and formulating the science of psychophysics, Fechner's assumptions have always been doubted. This is due to the fact that although he rigorously pursued the method of a quantitative psychology—the measurement of threshold levels, which is now a highly refined system based on mathematical calculations—this psychology was not considered by Fechner to be the end in itself which it has tended to become. Rather, it is evident by Fechner's very life that the object of psychophysics was to advocate a unitive point of view and a philosophy of a metaphysical or mystical nature. See also G. Stanley Hall, *Founders of Modern Psychology* (New York, 1912), pp. 125–77, who concludes, after observing and commenting on Fechner's work on the "after-life" problem and its relation to some kind of idea of Nirvana as a state of depth or infra-consciousness: "Some such sentiment as this, mystic but ineffably charming, seems to be the root of about all that this mystic prose-poet, seer, and scientist, the most Oriental perhaps of all Occidental minds, ever did and said. If so, to understand him we must ponder and find his relations with such men as Proclus, Plotinus, Böhme, and Eckhardt, but above all with the pundits and sages of Buddhistic India" (p. 174). Further emphasizing this aspect of Fechner's thought is Walter Lowrie, *Religion of a Scientist: Selections from Gustav Theodor Fechner* (New York, 1946), and of course there are the works of Fechner himself, including the *Comparative Anatomy of Angels*, a "humorous" account, written under the pseudonym of Dr. Mises in 1825, and *Zend Avesta* (Leipzig, 1851), and *Life After Death* (Chicago, 1945; first published in Leipzig, 1835).

Chapter Two

object, or objective knowledge? In a fundamental way Fechner's *Psychophysics* lays the groundwork for Bohr's law of
complementarity: the interaction of measuring instruments
(and, by extension, the measurer whom the measuring instruments reflect) and the objects measured forms an integral part of the whole phenomenon.[4] In a word, science has
come to realize the innate subjectivity of its own method:
the answers it creates/receives/discovers are only the pro-
jections of the creators/receivers/discoverers. Science as
method, to paraphrase Valéry, is part of a family of methods
or ways—an infinite group, all the elements of which we possess (unconsciously), consciousness of possession being the
secret of the inventors. If nothing else, Henry was acutely
aware of the nature of this inherent problem of science to
the point of seeking its resolution. His achievement must be
viewed in this respect, for Henry was indeed a precursor of
a system as startling in its unitive foundations as Descartes'
was in its dualistic assumption. Such indeed was the opinion
of no less eminent a person than Paul Valéry,[5] who saw in
Henry's work the creation of a system which was based on
theories of energy but whose ramifications reached to the
realms of culture and art.

Human history in all of its manifestations is not the accu-
mulation of "recorded events" nor a series of unconnected
happenings separated into categories each of which is gov-
erned by its own laws distinct in one ultimate way or another
from every other category. History is an elaborate equation
representing the development of consciousness on the human plane according to the laws of natural development or,
to use another term, evolution. The variable factors of the
equation are the various threads of human ideas and actions;

4. See, for instance, Niels Bohr, "Quantum Physics and Philosophy:
Causality and Complementarity, 1958," in *Essays 1958/1962 on Atomic
Physics and Human Knowledge* (London, 1962), pp. 1–7.
5. Paul Valéry, "Hommage à Henry," pp. 20–24.

Psychophysics in Perspective

innumerable as these are, all of them ultimately complement and balance one another. This view need not lead to either a deterministic, strictly causal and mechanistic interpretation or to a totally random interpretation of what is being considered. As quantum mechanics has indicated, the ultimate nature of the atom is not necessarily either a wave or a particle, but maybe, and perhaps more likely, both.

Whether such revolutionary turns of thought and method can ever be attributed to one man or idea is impossible to say; certain men or ideas may crystallize in themselves from a given perspective the necessary impetus for redirection. Such is the case with the idea of psychophysics as formulated by Fechner and pursued by Henry. In considering the physical and psychic states as corresponding attributes or functions of one another, Fechner formulated the paradigm for overcoming the dualistic schism in science and in Western culture in general. The original aim of psychophysics was neglected except by a few men like Henry, William James, and certain present-day researchers into the nature and extensibility of consciousness. On the other hand, psychophysics practiced as a traditional science is today *outer* psychophysics, and as such is almost wholly concerned with the most precise measurement of stimuli with reference to calculating threshold levels, largely ignoring the fact that Fechner conceived of an *inner* psychophysics as well as an *outer*. "However, there can be no development of outer psychophysics without constant regard to inner psychophysics, in view of the fact that the body's external world is functionally related to the mind only by the mediation of the body's internal world."[6] Psychophysics finally is a way of understanding reality as an integrated, interrelated whole. It is in this "tradition" that Henry pursued his "mathematics of the unconscious"[7] through the sensory portals of aesthetic experi-

6. Fechner, *Elements of Psychophysics*, 1:9.
7. This is a phrase used by Henry in the *Cercle chromatique* and the

17

ence in order to postulate his general law of psychomotor reactions by which states of consciousness could be determined, anticipated, and expanded.[8] It is in this same tradition that Jung states: "Now that the formerly hypostatised 'universal ideas' have turned out to be mental principles [inner psychophysics], it is dawning upon us to what an extent our whole experience of so-called reality is psychic; as a matter of fact, everything thought, felt, or perceived is a psychic image, and the world itself exists only so far as we are able to produce an image of it."[9]

Many conclusions and hypotheses have been drawn from this turn of affairs in modern science—a major departure from the classic point of view prevailing since the time of Descartes—and it is interesting how many of these conclusions suggest some relation to various other non-Western or even "primitive" modes of consciousness.[10] Since physics deals with matters basic to the physical or material nature of that universe upon which rests the entire weight of what Western civilization has come to term "the real," the effect of this revolutionary turn of events in psychology as well as

"L'Esthétique des formes," *Revue blanche* 7 (1894). Hericourt, "Une théorie mathématique," also emphasizes this aspect of Henry's thought. I shall develop this further in later chapters, particularly, 6.

8. This general law of psychomotor reactions could be said to be the theme of the *Cercle chromatique*. See also: Henry, "Sur une loi générale des réactions psychomotrices," *Revue philosophique* 30 (1890):107–11.

9. C. G. Jung, "Psychological Commentary," *The Tibetan Book of the Great Liberation,* ed. W. Y. Evans-Wentz (Oxford, 1954), p. 33.

10. McLuhan observes that nuclear physics tends to operate on the same assumptions about the universe as those used by the Taoists (*Understanding Media* [New York, 1964], p. 24). The works of Jung and Mircea Eliade also tend to develop this idea. See M. Eliade, *Cosmos and History* (New York, 1954), and *Myths, Dreams and Mysteries* (New York, 1960). Needless to say, even Bohr, "Quantum Physics and Philosophy," and Werner Heisenberg, *Physics and Philosophy* (New York, 1958), particularly the chapter, "The Role of Modern Physics in the Development of Human Thought," pp. 187–205, are aware of this development, or rather the consequences of this development in thought as a result of the conclusions of quantum mechanics and nuclear physics.

physics must ultimately manifest itself in an alteration of all aspects of the Western or technological consciousness whose basic tenets derive from a belief in the physical materiality of "reality."

Now, not only is it quite probable that, following from the vision of modern physics, humanity is in a process of merging into a new, more unified level of collective consciousness (this theme will be pursued later in this work), but in the equation of consciousness which comprises history—all that has "happened"—there are phases, periods, as in any other growth or natural development which complement and balance one another as they nourish themselves from what has been, give to one another in the "present," and nourish what is to come in the future. If this is so, it is not difficult, at least on a broad evolutionary level, to see in what we call the past an emerging pattern upon which are slowly becoming discernible the various stages in the development of consciousness. The turn of events in nineteenth-century psychology and twentieth-century physics is certainly a manifestation of one of the major junctures between stages of consciousness, and it will be our immediate purpose to trace the manner in which this juncture between stages in the development of consciousness has manifested itself in the realm of art and aesthetics.

In what way has Western art and aesthetics manifested the change in modes of consciousness now becoming so clearly revealed in science and already so obvious in technology? The question is not as general as it sounds, for, indeed, much change and "revolution" have revealed themselves stylistically and even technologically in the art fashions of the last one hundred years or so. But in all of the parade of "isms" where is to be found the lead thread, the thread with which the new consciousness will weave the cloth of its vision? In view of all that has been said or discussed thus far, with particular reference to recent Western science, it seems wise to

Chapter Two

consider, first of all, the origins of the particular thread contemporaneous with the rise of psychophysics in the late nineteenth century.

As in the late fifteenth and early sixteenth centuries, there occurred in the late nineteenth and early twentieth centuries a cross-fertilization of the arts and, in the broadest sense of the word, the sciences, whether philosophical, physical, or psychological. The result in both cases was the emergence of a new mode of visual perception and the decline of the preceding mode. After Fechner's *Elements of Psychophysics*, came the works of Helmholtz and Wundt, forming the core of classical psychophysical literature and research.[11] All of this work deals with the nature of psychosensory experience, and it need only be stated here that never before in the history of the West had there been a time when so much research was being carried out in this particular domain—that of sense experience and consciousness. Emphasis on the nature of perception and not on its *object*—the "matter" of classical science—had its artistic expression in the entire phenomenon of "impressionism." Herein lies the significance of impressionism as a revolutionary event. How conscious a man like Monet was of this significance is not clear. At least it can be said that Monet's art was the "unconscious" and synchronous expression of the psychophysical turn of events in the 1860s and 1870s. By the 1880s, however, psychophysics was an important intellectual and cultural current, and its effect upon the arts was of a *conscious* nature.

11. Perhaps most important is the work of H. L. F. von Helmholtz whose *Handbuch der Physiologischen Optik* (Leipzig, 1855–66) and *Popular Lectures* (New York, 1881), are an absolute essential in understanding the phenomena of impressionism within the context of nineteenth-century science. According to Herrnstein and Boring, *A Source-Book in the History of Psychology* (Cambridge, 1965), Wilhelm Wundt (1832–1920) "was the elementist *par excellence*. For him psychology studies the mental elements (sensations, images, feelings) and their combinations into *Vorstellungen* (perceptions, ideas)," p. 399. See also, Hall, *Modern Psychology*, pp. 247–308, for a genial assessment of Helmholtz, and pp. 311–458 for one of Wundt.

Psychophysics in Perspective

In France, during the 1880s, psychophysics and psychology in general, the study of the psychic aspect of human experience, was a subject of great debate and popularity. In 1883, Delboeuf published his study of psychophysics.[12] Volumes of the *Revue philosophique* for the years 1889–90 carried a large number of articles on problems of sensation, perception, and related psychological matters: vision, hypnotism, automatism, and so on. Also in a series of issues of the *Revue philosophique* of this period there is an interesting discussion of the problem of psychophysics and aesthetics, including an exchange of letters between G. Sorel and Charles Henry over an article on Henry's research by George Lachalas published late in 1889 in the same journal.[13] Finally, in addition to the opening of the International Congress of Physiological Psychology in Paris in 1889, an event occurring in the midst of Henry's aesthetic investigations, one might mention the publication of Henri Bergson's *Essai sur les données immédiates*

12. J. R. L. Delboeuf, *Examen critique de la loi psychophysique: sa base et sa signification* (Paris, 1883). See also Herrnstein and Boring, *A Source-Book*, pp. 79–81.

13. See G. Lachelas, "Le *Cercle chromatique* et le *Rapporteur esthétique* de Charles Henry," *Revue philosophique*, 28 (1889):635–45. See also G. Sorel, "Contributions psycho-physique à l'esthétique," "Esthétique et psycho-physique," *Revue philosophique* 29 (1889):561–79 and 181–84 respectively; idem, "Contributions psychophysiques à l'étude esthétique," *Revue philosophique* 30:22–41; also, Charles Henry, "Esthétique et psychophysique," *Revue philosophique* 29:332–36, in reply. Sorel's criticism of Henry is fundamental. For example, Sorel cannot conceive psychophysics as universal law as Henry does, but only as a series of multiple laws. Nor does Sorel see any necessary relation between music and the other arts. Contrary to Henry, he does not view pleasure as an element of aesthetic emotion, and he does not understand how the principle of dynamogeny and inhibition can be at the base of an aesthetic doctrine. The only use Sorel can see for psychophysics in aesthetics is in the study of modern metallic constructions. Lachelas is scarcely more sympathetic, and like Sorel is skeptical of any attempt at posing the aesthetic problem under the form of a synthesis. Henry's reply to Sorel is most polite, as he asks him to utilize one of the aesthetic instruments such as the aesthetic protractor. Also in the *Revue philosophique* 29:445–48, in conjunction with the meeting of the Société de psychologie physiologique is "Projet de questionnaire psycho-physique," by J. Hericourt.

de la conscience, also of the same year.[14] In many ways Bergson and Henry cover the same territory. Bergson acknowledges psychophysics, but with the qualification, which in retrospect seems more semantic than substantive, that "the mistake Fechner made . . . was that he believed in an interval between two successive sensations S and S', when there is simply a *passing* from one to the other and not a *difference* in the arithmetical sense of the word."[15] Bergson sees psychophysics as pushing to the extreme the "fundamental but natural mistake of regarding sensation as magnitudes."[16] Whether this is a "natural mistake" is open to question; on the other hand, in distinguishing himself from the psychophysicists, Bergson loses sight of common ground he shares with them: the basic subjectivity of all experience. Stimulus may indeed be measured, but stimulus is only the outer aspect of consciousness; the inner aspect dealing with immeasurable subjective states and their corresponding motor reflexes is another matter.

In this respect Charles Henry may indeed be viewed as the inner psychophysicist par excellence. Not confining himself to mere observation and laboratory experiments, Henry relentlessly applied his conclusions to all facets of contemporary life and acquainted himself with some of the leading artistic personalities of his time, a fact which not only rounds out the character of this "scientist," but also lends to his personality a rather unique quality. To further fill out a picture of Henry the symbolist psychophysiologist, let me quote a

14. Translated as *Time and Free Will* (New York, 1960).
15. Ibid., pp. 67–68.
16. Ibid., p. 70. In his discussion of psychophysics, Bergson takes into account the work of Delboeuf and Fechner, but there is no mention of Henry. Bergson seems to object to the mathematizing, as he sees it, of subjective phenomena or, rather, of the differences between two given subjective phenomena or states. In his words, "as soon as it is proved that two sensations can be equal without being identical, psychophysics will be established. But it is this equality which seems to me open to question" (p. 57). For Henry it is not so much a question of equality as complementarity. See below, chapter 6.

Psychophysics in Perspective

thumbnail biography by the critic, anarchist, and honorary 'pataphysician, actually 'patacessor,[17] Félix Fénéon:

> Charles Henry in 1886 declares without flinching in an esthetic article: "Rhythm is a determining change of direction on a circumference whose center is the center of change, a geometric division possible in the terms of Gauss' theory."
>
> Measures with a dynamograph the value of a metaphor by Mallarmé, comments on the blackboard on the verse of Jules Laforgue, reduces to equations a painting by Degas. Would prove the rigorous relations between the solubility of lead nitrate and the Taiping Rebellion.[18]

Bearing out this characterization of Henry is a statement recorded some eight years later in 1894, by Paul Signac:

> Charles Henry came to see me. He is getting to be more poetical. He will start from an exact and scientific premise, and from it he will draw the most delightfully whimsical conclusions. Then he tries to find mathematical proofs for them. . . .[19]

This whimsical aspect of Henry is still evident in the latter and less-known half of his life. One writer quotes Henry's views on death: "It is only after death that I shall commence to amuse myself."[20] And to round off this initial consideration of Henry the symbolist psychophysicist, another author in the *Hommage à Henry* relays Henry's thought that "You cannot

17. See, for instance, "The 'Patacessors," pt. 2 of "What Is 'Pataphysics?," *Evergreen Review* 4, no. 13 (May–June, 1960):103–5.

18. In Félix Fénéon, *Oeuvres* (Paris, 1948), p. 200. After Henry's death Fénéon published an article on him in *Bulletin de la vie artistique* (November 15, 1926).

19. Paul Signac, "Journaux inédits," published and edited by John Rewald, *Gazette des beaux arts* (July–September, 1949), p. 98. Entry for December 14, 1894.

20. Quoted in Juliette Roche, "Hommage à Henry," p. 31. Also with regard to this general area of research, Henry published at least two articles, "Ce que je sais de dieu," *Cahiers contemporains* 1 (1925), and "Vie et Survie," *Cahiers contemporains* 2 (1926). On this matter, Henry has much in common with Gustav Fechner.

23

Chapter Two

make mathematics if you are not a poet, otherwise you are merely an imbecile."[21] Indeed, it should be remembered that to the first edition of the important symbolist journal *La vogue*, which he also helped to found, Henry contributed a prose poem entitled "Vision."[22]

Henry died a solitary figure, unmarried, and without any apparent disciples, leaving behind a bibliography which suggests a mentality that is at once restless and aloofly erudite, a blend of Valéry's Monsieur Teste, Jarry's Faustroll, and Lewis Carroll. Still, there is a logic to Charles Henry's psychophysics which suggests a system of integral wholeness. According to Paul Valéry, in whose work and thought there are, as shall be seen, reflections of Henry's method, Charles Henry began to realize the synthesis of the various fields of knowledge—science and art—as *energy*.[23] A figure like Valéry's M. Teste, who "had discovered laws of the mind that we know nothing of,"[24] Charles Henry and his work remain largely unnoticed except as a curious intrusion into art history—in its own way a justly 'pataphysical fate. Perhaps, like the "mystical art" that Henry predicted for the not too distant future, the proper decipherment of his method remains for an age more perfectly practiced in the science of the mind. Mysticism in Henry's terms

21. Quoted in Fernand Divoire, "Hommage à Henry," p. 34.
22. I have not had a chance to see "Vision." In a letter to Gustave Kahn, dated April 23, 1886, Laforgue comments, "Tell Henry that I have been disconcerted by his "Vision." There is too much in it and yet it ends as too little—the end is the best: the verticals, the violet of the vest-lining. But what are we to make of the sudden entrance of the company of the *Meistersingers!* These folk who arrive as provincial orphans with their talking banners, their *foot-wear, their caps, their attributes of Vulcan,* etc. . . . all the crafts represented, there's nothing to see in this Eldorado. A volume where Henry would place his artificial paradises [*paradis artificiels;* see Baudelaire's book of the same name concerning his drug experience] in realized visions—that will be a very curious breviary. But this vision leaves me cold, and it is not thought through enough" (Jules Laforgue, *Lettres à un ami* [Paris, 1941], p. 176). Henry's vision would seem to be mystical, utopian, and unliterary!
23. Valéry, "Hommage à Henry," p. 21.
24. Valéry, *Selected Writings,* p. 237.

24

can be considered the deployment of biopsychic energy according to cosmic laws; indeed, to reveal the way in which this occurs within the individual is the function which Henry ascribes to psychotherapy, thus suggesting an affinity with Jung's psychology of the unconscious. The comparison is worth pursuing, if one considers the archetypes as manifestations of cosmic principles or law.[25]

Certainly in view of even the brief remarks made thus far, Henry's thought merits an evaluation and understanding that will endeavor to reveal the method which moved his mind to consider the diversity of topics upon which he worked as manifestations of an all-embracing principle. Fechner, the founder of modern experimental psychology—psychophysics as he called it—worked under such a principle, which operated as something which could be alternatively and/or simultaneously called night view (materialism) and day view (mysticism).[26] Scholars or scientists adhering to the night view of materialism are naturally skeptical of Fechner's day view, even though it is obvious that development of the day view, or at least acknowledgment of the two complementary views, was Fechner's avowed aim. Fechner issued "seven calls" to the sleeping public, which he saw as being totally caught up in the night view. Though he did not overtly proselytize, much the same holds true for Henry, whose philosophy of complementaries was even more unified, though perhaps more abstrusely stated than Fechner's. Here again it is worth recalling Kuhn's notion that the real revolutionary break-

25. The reader is again referred to Henry's *Théorie du rayonnement,* in which Henry most fully elaborates these principles as electromagnetic, gravitational, and biopsychic resonators; the resonator is not to be understood as a specific material phenomenon—indeed one does not speak of matter—but as a *function.* Therapy is then the reestablishment of auto-regulation to the biopsychic resonator by making into a conscious process what was an unconscious impulse (see, specifically, p. 102).

26. See above, n. 3. Fechner issued seven "calls" in the form of books more popularly addressed than his more rigorously scientific studies; the most notable of these was the *Zend Avesta* of 1851. See also Lowrie, *Religion of a Scientist.*

throughs in science go unnoticed or even scoffed at and are naturally considered unscientific or eccentric and inapplicable precisely because they presuppose a mode of perception other than that which predominates at the time of the breakthrough.[27]

Henry was obviously very aware that there was no real development in science without a complementary development in the subjective consideration of those things which fall under the domain of art. As he wrote in 1889, "certain phenomena which, for ourselves, are the affair of consciousness were unconscious at an epoch as near to our own as the Greco-Roman. Human beings are, therefore, incontestably progressing towards a state of ever greater life enhancement."[28] This statement should not be understood as an expression of nineteenth-century materialistic positivism; Henry is obviously talking about consciousness as an evolutionary phenomenon, whose end is "greater life enhancement." Here Henry begs comparison with Bergson or, even more recently, Teilhard de Chardin, whose theory of the evolution of consciousness is one of the most accepted in terms of traditional Western scientific thought.[29]

Henry, familiar with the origin of classic Western science in the seventeenth century, a subject that shall be taken up shortly, was able to view the events of his time with a certain amount of perspective; certainly his emphasis on synthesis is in one way an answer to the Cartesian division of phenomena into the objective and subjective, a view in which the "observer" is necessarily distinct from the phenomena he is observing. One might even consider the "romanticism" of the nineteenth century and the various "irrational" art movements of the twentieth century, as aspects of "Cartesian fall-

27. See above, chapter 1, n. 6.
28. Charles Henry, "Contraste, rythme, et mesure," *Revue philosophique* 28:356ff. Also quoted in J. Russell, *Seurat* (London, 1965), pp. 191–92.
29. I have in mind particularly Teilhard de Chardin, *The Phenomenon of Man* (New York, 1959).

out," representing a balance of the equation of Western consciousness, which has laid such a great stress on "objectivity." And thus Henry could say:

> I do not believe in the future . . . of naturalism, or in general of any realistic school. On the contrary, I believe in the more or less imminent advent of a very idealistic and even mystic art based on new techniques. I believe this because we are witnessing a greater and greater development and diffusion of scientific methods and industrial efforts; the economic future of all nations is involved in it and social questions force us to follow this lead, for, after all, the problem of the progressive life of all peoples can be summed up thus: *produce much, cheaply, and in a very short time.* Europe is obliged not to let itself be annihilated or even outrun by America, which has for a very long time combined its national education and its entire organization for the purpose of reaching this goal. I believe in the future of an art which would be the reverse of any ordinary logical or historical method, precisely because our intellects, exhausted by purely rational efforts, will feel the need to refresh themselves with entirely opposite states of mind.[30]

Lest he be misunderstood with regard to mysticism or idealism, Henry adds, "You have only to look at this singular vogue of occult, spiritualist and other doctrines, which are false because they can satisfy neither reason nor imagination."[31]

This entire statement, so rich and suggestive, can be taken as the basis for many of the speculative ideas presented herein, particularly with regard to the artistic or aesthetic developments of the twentieth century; it also provides insight into how Henry might have viewed that art movement which reflected so many of his own ideas and principles,

---

30. Quoted in Rewald, *Post-impressionism*, p. 483, from *L'écho de Paris* (June, 1891). See also Camillo Pissarro's comment in *Lettres à son fils* (Paris, 1950), p. 256.
31. Rewald, *Post-impressionism*, p. 483.

neo-impressionism. Indeed, given this statement made in 1891 by the scientific guide of this movement, it is imperative to reconsider the nature and limitations of the first *consciously* psychophysical art venture in history. It is possible that, Seurat's death not withstanding, neo-impressionism at the historical moment it appeared could have gone no further than the amusing but somewhat forced *Portrait of Fénéon,* by Signac, precisely because the proper idealistic and mystic mind was nowhere in sight to fulfill the profound possibilities suggested by a psychophysical aesthetic. On the other hand, given Henry's influence, it is reasonable to assume that the general phenomenon of art nouveau, for instance, is more precisely psychophysical in its aesthetic assumptions than has yet been considered.

In sum, without becoming involved in technicalities, let it be said that psychophysics is a science whose object of study is the nature of sense experience; as such, the works of Helmholtz and Wundt can be considered as "classics" of psychophysics.[32] However, because the underlying assumption of psychophysics as originally conceived is that matter is a function of consciousness as much as consciousness is a function of matter, an idea thoroughly against the grain of traditional Cartesian science, there developed, naturally enough, a reaction to the very word "psychophysics," to say nothing of the philosophical assumption which underlay it.[33] The chief merit or significance of psychophysics, however, is that it

32. See above, n. 11.
33. This is clear from the assumptions of Herrnstein and Boring, *A Source-Book.* See also E. G. Boring, *The Physical Dimensions of Consciousness* (New York, 1933), in which the writer eschews any idea of an impalpable or imponderable consciousness; indeed with the development of behavioralism early in the twentieth century the *psychic* aspect of psychology tends to go into eclipse, at least with regard to "official" psychology. Much of what the nineteenth-century psychophysicist studied is now in the realm of parapsychology—that realm which deals most specifically with the psychic phenomena which quantitative and behavioral psychology scarcely acknowledges. E. R. Jaensch, *Eidetic Images* (London, 1930) deals with the problem and strikes an interesting middle ground (p. 35).

Psychophysics in Perspective

shifts the object of research from the investigation of matter to the "representation"[34] of the idea of matter in our sense experience, a shift whose ramifications are yet to be properly assessed.

In this historical development, Henry's work is first of all very much in the tradition of Fechner with regard to the unitive assumption that matter is an attribute of consciousness. Secondly, because this science is the study of sense nature, much of Henry's early psychophysical research turned to the realm of aesthetics, something even Fechner turned to in the 1870s.[35] And finally, because Henry so well realized the revolutionary nature of the function and importance of psychophysics in the general development of thought, he turned to a reassessment of the models upon which traditional thought is based. It is this aspect of Henry that shall next be considered.

34. Indeed Henry defines matter as "*that which is directed* in our representations," and representation is defined as "every expression, more or less motor, conscious or not, of an idea, abstract or concrete" (*Cercle chromatique*, p. 164). Matter is then considered a psychic function; again this invites comparison with Govinda, *Early Buddhist Philosophy*, who states that in consequence of the Buddhist psychological attitude the field of research is not the investigation of the essence of matter, "but only into the essence of the sense-perceptions and experiences that create in us the *representation* or idea of matter" (emphasis added).

35. Gustav Fechner, *Vorschule der Aesthetik* (Leipzig, 1876). See also Richter, *Perspectives in Aesthetics,* pp. 286–93. Needless to say, Fechner sought to create a general and universal aesthetics which would combine the view from "above," which begins with the most general ideas, with the view from "below," which proceeds from the more empirical particulars. Henry's aesthetic system is such a one, combining as it does views from above—the mystic, Pythagorean side of Henry—with those from below—the Cartesian, empirical side.

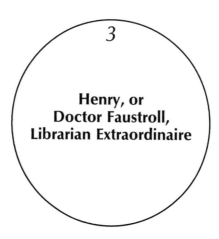

3

Henry, or
Doctor Faustroll,
Librarian Extraordinaire

D OCTOR Faustroll is the 'pataphysical hero of what Alfred Jarry called a "neo-scientific novel," the *Gestes
et opinions du docteur Faustroll, 'pataphysicien*, published in
1911, the year in which Charles Henry, Director of the Laboratory of the Physiology of Sensations at the Sorbonne, read
his paper (actually part of his thesis) on memory and habit
before the section of artistic psychology of the General Psychology Institute. One writer describes the situation by stating that Henry's "colleagues remained silent and baffled, understanding nothing of his mathematical juggling which was
of such an extraordinary transcendence."[1] Indeed there is
more than a little of the 'pataphysical in Henry's relentless
pursuit of what Goloubew calls a mathematical and experimental aesthetic.[2] And there is more than a little of Doctor

1. René Doyen, "Hommage à Henry," p. 37.
2. Victor Goloubew, in his introduction to Charles Henry, *Mémoire et
habitude* (Paris, 1911). "In sum," Henry writes, "memory is characterized
by the evolution of representations towards a state that is more and more
complete; habit is characterized by the evolution of the duration of a
complete representation towards durations of ever smaller establishment,
tending asymptomatically towards a limit" (p. 2). Obviously memory tends
to states of heightened sensitivity, habit to insensitivity, which—not to
confuse it with fatigue—we can call adaptation. For Henry memory, habit,
and adaptation "constitute three irreducible biological properties which
are all functions of sensation and of a conscious or unconscious sensitivity

Henry, or Doctor Faustroll

Faustroll—even of Faust—in Henry, as several of his biographers have described him:[3] the man whose aim was to establish, among other things, the importance of the laws of sensation with regard to the study of art. It is well to recall here the aims of 'pataphysics as described in *Faustroll:*

['Pataphysics] is the science of the particular, despite the common opinion that the only science is that of the general. 'Pataphysics will examine the laws governing exceptions, and will explain the universe supplementary to this one; or, less ambitiously, will describe a universe that can be envisaged in the place of the traditional one, since the laws that are supposed to have been discovered in the traditional universe are also correlations of exceptions, albeit more frequent ones, but in any case accidental data which, reduced to the status of unexceptional exceptions, possess no longer even the virtue of originality.[4]

Jarry's definition is as incisive a critique of traditional science as has been made; and certainly Henry's multiple intel-

---

in relation to time. These terms are rigorously defined, in the case of consciousness by psychophysics, and in the case of unconsciousness and in general, by psychobiological energy" (p. 3). The first part of Henry's thesis is *Sensation et énergie* (Paris, 1910), in which he states: "as nutrition and embryological development are conditioned by special irritabilities, and as all the irritabilities are at every moment the function of one another, one can envision the ensemble of the phenomena of life from the point of view of irritability and seek to define this property by the mathematical function which relates the reactions to the excitant, to the length of the excitation, and to the amount of energy expended." Needless to say, for Henry, sensation is the sole reality. It is also well to keep in mind that Henri Bergson wrote on the same subject, more or less, publishing in 1896 *Matière et mémoire* (English edition, *Matter and Memory,* New York, 1959). Bergson's position is not as extreme as Henry's, or rather Bergson tries to steer a middle course, preserving the reality of both matter and mind.

3. In "Hommage à Henry," Juliette Roche, Gustave Kahn, and even Paul Signac have similar descriptions of Henry. Mme Roche describes Henry as "très docteur Faust" (p. 30) wearing his fantastic great-coat in his garden on a barren day in March.

4. Alfred Jarry, *Selected Writings,* ed. Roger Shattuck (New York, 1965).

lectual endeavors can be said to have the same aim: to explain the universe supplementary to this one, or, at least, to envisage one in the place of the traditional universe. This Henry did in a manner similar to the 'pataphysician, by studying the laws which govern the particulars of sensation and sense phenomena. As one writer points out, Henry combated the traditional (scientific) system with its own arms: "by scrupulous experiments, with the balance of precision, test-tube and microscope, he demonstrated the inanity of the experience [of scientific materialism]."[5] In fact, with this idea in mind it becomes easy to discern in Henry's career and life a pattern which leads up to this final conclusion; a survey of Henry's special interests are like the piecing together of the collective psyche of the West. By the end of his life Henry had indeed completed his vision of a universe supplementary to this one.

Charles Singer states:

> It is no accident that, precisely during these two centuries (1700–1900), certain kinds of "philosophical inquiries"—as Newton and his contemporaries always described their labors—came gradually to be known as "scientific researches." Science, the knowledge of nature, was separated from philosophy, the search for the key to the universe. The change represented a fragmentation of interests that has lasted beyond the period we are considering [1900]. For this reason, among others, it is peculiarly difficult to present the history of modern science as a coherent whole, but only a bit at a time, each science choosing its own bit. This departmentalism becomes increasingly self-conscious.[6]

When Henry began his investigation in the 1870s as a pupil of the famous experimental physician, Claude Bernard, it was as if he had been aware of this observation concerning the

5. Roche, "Hommage à Henry," p. 26.
6. Charles Singer, *A Short History of Scientific Ideas to 1900* (Oxford, 1959), p. 297.

Henry, or Doctor Faustroll

departmentalization and fragmentation of science and, by extension, of all knowledge since the time of Newton. From the start, it can be said, Henry's aim was to repair this state of fragmentation by envisaging a new universe whose laws were unified, affecting all disciplines and "sciences" equally. As has already been observed, Henry's technique was to use the very tools and methods that were both the cause and the effect of the fragmented situation: scientific method, mathematical proof, publication of historical data and documentation.

It is essential to realize the importance of this idea for two reasons: first, because the practice and study of art are naturally a part of the fragmentation of Western consciousness in the very ways that the interests and purposes of art have been defined and pursued. Secondly, because in the way and end of Henry's universal vision there is the understanding that an aesthetic and even a historical development have occurred. But aesthetics and the historical development as well as the very nature of art are not to be studied in a way that emphasizes the separateness of art, but in a way which relates the aesthetic phenomena to the organism as a whole. Aesthetics and the history of art, following Henry's research and example, are most properly studied and understood as an aspect of historical psychology, in the case of art history, and as applied psychophysics, in the case of practice.

With unerring instinct Henry went to the heart of the problem. Basing himself on a thorough knowledge of mathematics, which led him naturally enough to studies of the history of science, with particular reference to the origins of "science" in the seventeenth century, Henry was able to address himself through mathematics and historical method to the source of the problem about which Charles Singer wrote in his *History of Scientific Ideas:* the fragmentation of knowledge. It is well to note that Henry's approach from the beginning was a synthesizing one: mathematical interest combined with historical method. It is not at all surprising that Henry's

33

Chapter Three

first publication should have been *Sur l'origine de la convention dite de Descartes* (1878).[7] For it was finally the dualism underlying the whole Cartesian system—the system of modern science exemplified by Newton—that Henry sought to refute, precisely by using Descartes' methods, or those derived from that method.[8] W. C. Dampier writes: "Thus Descartes was the first to formulate complete dualism, that sharp distinction between soul and body, mind and matter, which

7. This is a most interesting discourse on the origin of the convention used by Descartes in the formulation of the theory of coordinates. This convention is a sign—V—which Henry finally traces to an Etruscan origin, but not without displaying an amazing wealth of knowledge concerning Egyptian, Phoenician, and Chinese systems of mathematical notation. Henry concludes that "the honor of this conception belongs to a collective activity and not to an historical individuality [that is, Descartes]" (*Revue archéologique* 35:251–59).

With regard to Henry's involvement with Descartes and the entire Cartesian system, it is also interesting to note that, in a brief article on Descartes, Paul Valéry wrote: "Then he [Descartes] proceeds to invent a Universe and an animal and imagines that he explains them. Whatever his delusions in this direction may be, his efforts have been of the greatest consequence. That is my second point. Even if the Cartesian universe has suffered the same fate as all the conceived or conceivable universes, nevertheless the world in which our 'civilization' lives still bears the marks of the way and manner of thinking of which I have spoken.

"This world is imbued with applications of mathematical standards. Our lives are more regulated according to mathematical principles, and everything which escapes representation by numbers, all knowledge that cannot be measured, is judged with depreciation. The word 'Knowledge' is increasingly denied to anything which cannot be translated into figures" (*Selected Writings*, p. 205). A most interesting observation, considering Henry's own efforts.

8. It is interesting to recall Blake's depiction of Newton measuring infinity at the bottom of the Great Ocean as representative of the degradation of consciousness; Newton, in this view, would be at the peripheral limit of individual self-consciousness. Also within this context, we can view Henry's effort as a part of the reorientation of consciousness towards its own integration and self-fulfillment, that is, away from fragmented, individual self-consciousness and towards renewed contact with its own depths, its own roots, its own source.

On the other hand, it is also well to keep in mind that Newton was an alchemist, and was closer to Blake than Blake might have imagined. As Henry was later aware, it was the work of the savants and intellectuals

afterwards became so general a belief and so important a philosophy."[9] Henry was most certainly aware of this aspect of Descartes' thought, and of the implications of this thought in the fragmentation of the various scientific disciplines as they presented themselves in Henry's day. To overcome the dualism, Henry, like Fechner, turned the scientific method to the study of sensations or, more precisely, to the mathematical measurement of sensations.

Curiously enough, Henry's second publication, "Sur une première rédaction du *Traité de la connaissance de Dieu et de soi-même* de Bossuet" (1878), was in direct contrast to his study on Descartes. Bossuet was a contemporary and fellow countryman of Pascal and Descartes, and of a persuasion similar to Pascal's.[10] This publication was in the time of Henry's student days, when he was studying rather freely Sanskrit, German, and the history of literature in the Bibliothèque nationale, where he met various young friends, among them Gustave Kahn and Jules Laforgue.

But at first, pursuing the initial studies of the origins of classical Western science, Henry turned his attention to mathematics, for the language of mathematics is the language

---

after Newton who "dethroned" alchemy, astrology, and the traditional sciences which had fallen into a state of such great disrepute and which Henry felt called upon to rehabilitate, but in terms of *current* knowledge, that is, radiation and quantum theory. Henry is, without qualification, a modern alchemist.

9. W. C. Dampier, *A History of Science and Its Relation to Philosophy and Religion* (Cambridge, Eng., 1966 [1st ed., 1929]), p. 136. I have found this book invaluable, and the author's viewpoint both broad and sensitive.

10. Bossuet (1627–1704) was one of the more outstanding clerical figures of France in the seventeenth century. Friend of Fénélon and St. Vincent de Paul and correspondent with Leibnitz, as well as tutor to the Dauphin, Bossuet excited the imagination of Paul Valéry, who found in him a writer who stands above all others: "He is essentially calculating, as are all those who are called *classic*. He proceeds by construction, while we proceed by accident; he gambles on the expectation he creates, while the moderns gamble on surprise" (Valéry, *Selected Writings*, p. 206). Henry's historical taste is impeccable!

which this science respects. By mastering mathematics and applying it to all branches of Cartesian science, Henry, once again following Fechner, sought to discover the mathematical relationships governing *all* human understanding. It is important to grasp this, for Henry's life developed in definite stages, each being a preparation for the next, and the whole being an example of the putting into practice of what we may call the principles of an evolutionary psychology. There followed a series of mathematical treatises, all published in 1879, whose titles and general content are of necessity in line with Henry's development:

"Sur l'origine de quelques notations mathématiques."[11]

"Opusculum de Multiplicatione et Divisione Sexagesimalibus Diophanto vel Pappo attribuendum primo editione."[12]

"Sur une valeur approchée de $\sqrt{2}$ et sur deux approximations de $\sqrt{3}$."[13]

These precise studies gave Henry the operational base he needed for his later series of lectures on the mathematical laws of sensation.[14] These early mathematical studies were followed, still in 1879, by the publication of letters of Ma-

11. *Revue archéologique* 37 (1878):324–33. This again is an amazing little article displaying an erudition which is without parallel. Taking the sign of "zero," as well as all the various mathematical signs—those for plus, minus, multiplication, division, infinity, and so on—and tracing them through the various cultures in which these signs have operated—Greek, Egyptian, Indian, Arabic—provides Henry a perfect vehicle, as it were, for conversing with certain historical figures. Among these are such mathematicians as Archimedes and Pythagoras, the alchemist Fludd and the Arab master of algebra, Al-Kharizmi, as well as such a lesser-known figure as Balthazar Monconys, the seventeenth-century traveler. In the second part of this study (*Revue archéologique* 38:1–10), Henry discusses the sign for infinity, tracing it through Hebrew, Chinese, and Tibetan accounts, and concludes this article with some observations on the origin of the zodiac in Chaldea and of the signs of the planets pertaining to this zodiac.

12. Halis Saxioniae: H. W. Schmitt (1879). Diophantus was a celebrated Greek mathematician from Alexandria who lived some time in the third or fourth century A.D. and is often credited with the invention of algebra.

13. *Bulletin des sciences mathématiques* (1879).

14. Georges Bohn, "Hommage à Henry," p. 73, recalls, from probably around 1900, Henry's lectures on the "mathematical laws of sensations."

Henry, or Doctor Faustroll

dame Lafayette, of Bossuet, and of Flechier;[15] also in 1879 Henry published new documents on Huygens and Roberval, thus extending his knowledge of the scientific culture of the seventeenth century.[16] These publications are most crucial, for in them the very founders and inventors of both the ideas and the instruments of modern science discuss, often tentatively, their preliminary observations, particularly with regard to other modes of knowledge such as astrology or alchemy; ultimately the new science managed to banish these other modes into the realm of the unpardonably superstitious, not totally without reason, and yet in a manner so dogmatic as to be irrational.[17]

Mention is made of this relation between what came to be called science and disciplines like astrology or alchemy because Henry himself was aware that in the fundamental understanding of the so-called prescientific modes of thought there was a stratum of awareness which modern science, in all its fragmented disparateness, could well employ; this was the understanding of the cosmos as a totally interrelated and interdependent unity. Indeed, in his great summary work, *Essai de généralisation de la théorie du rayonnement*, Henry touches on an idea of Kepler's concerning the equilibrium of the gravitational masses of the planets and the sun with those masses which Henry called biological: "For all of these gravitational masses one can draw η nervous correspondences. All of this leads to a rehabilitation of astrology, which distinguished scholars once cultivated, for it led them to practical

15. *Un érudit homme du monde, homme d'église, homme de cour: lettres inédites de Madame de Lafayette, de Bossuet, de Flechier, etc.* (Paris, 1878). Henry's fascination is revealed by the title of this work, the first of many letters and memoirs that he was to edit.

16. Charles Henry, *Huygens et Roberval, documents nouveaux* (Leyden: E. J. Brill, 1879).

17. This is borne out in an exchange of letters between Huygens and Roberval, the latter a French mathematician, concerning a lady whom Huygens met and who wished to have her horoscope charted. Huygens states that he has no belief in the business, but sends the lady's natal information on to Roberval, who apparently does (ibid., p. 26).

results conforming to experience."[18] Henry goes on to state how this science, astrology, was wrongly condemned in the seventeenth century due to *incomplete knowledge*. This condemnation was then taken up by the intellectuals as dogma.[19]

Here it is well to regard the reflections of the 1945 Nobel Prize winner in physics, W. Pauli, also writing about the ideas of Kepler, seventeenth-century science, and alchemy:

> It is obviously out of the question for modern man to revert to the archaistic point of view that paid the price of its unity and completeness by a naive ignorance of nature. His strong desire for unification of his world view, however, impels him to recognize the significance of the prescientific stage of knowledge from the development of scientific ideas . . . by supplementing the investigation of this knowledge, directed inward. The former process is devoted to adjusting our knowledge to external objects; the latter should bring to light the archetypal images used in the creation of our scientific concepts. *Only by combining both these directions of research may complete understanding be obtained.* [Emphasis added.]
>
> Among scientists in particular, the universal desire for a greater unification of the world view is greatly intensified by the fact that, though we now have natural sciences, we no longer have a total scientific picture of the world. Since the discovery of the quantum of action, physics has gradually been forced to relinquish its proud claim to be able to understand, in principle, the *whole* world. This very circumstance, however, as a correction of earlier one-sidedness, could contain the germ of progress toward a unified conception of the entire cosmos of which the natural sciences are only a part.[20]

18. Henry, *Théorie du rayonnement,* p. 94.
19. Ibid.
20. W. Pauli, "The Influence of Archetypal Ideas on the Scientific Theories of Kepler," in *The Interpretation of Nature and the Psyche* (New York, 1955), pp. 208–9. This work also contains the essay by C. G. Jung, "Synchronicity: An Acausal Connecting Principle." What better example of psychophysical research than the two essays in this book?

Henry, or Doctor Faustroll

Henry's psychophysical conception is in many ways such a science or unified theory which, though little known now, did have a certain popularity in the later nineteenth century. One reason little has been heard or known of Henry is that, as several of the biographers in the *Hommage à Henry* note, the last years of his life were darkened by the systematic opposition of official scholars.[21] Certain nineteenth-century individuals, taking cognizance of the state of scientific knowledge and its assumptions, were already laying the groundwork for an all-encompassing system which, though partially recognized, soon met increasing resistance, only to be vindicated by the discoveries of men like Pauli, Max Planck, Niels Bohr, and Werner Heisenberg, not to mention the efforts of men like C. G. Jung. It may well be that the system formulated by the nineteenth-century psychophysicists will bear the same relation to the development of future thought and cultural/social institutions as the science of the seventeenth century bears to the present. Only through such an understanding is one able to begin to have a true estimate of the importance or place of psychophysics and the developmental nature of Henry's thought. If seventeenth-century science demonstrated the folly of those alchemists who took literally the idea of the elemental importance of the philosopher's stone, of quicksilver, or of the transmutation of gross substance into gold, so the discovery in the late nineteenth and early twentieth centuries of electricity and electromagnetism, of the interchangeability of energy and the endlessly transformable nature of matter, demonstrates the folly of scientific materialism pursued as the ultimate doctrine of "objec-

21. See, for instance, Bohn, "Hommage à Henry," p. 77. Apparently Henry was pressured out of his laboratory at the Sorbonne and, in the years 1924–25, set up his laboratory at Coyes near Versailles. Resistance was most strongly addressed to Henry's work on the hydrogen "catalyst" as well as to his work on the resonators—electromagnetic, gravitational, and biopsychic. Indeed, Henry was always terribly difficult to fit into any niche and the position he held at the Sorbonne—Director of the Laboratory of the Physiology of Sensations—was created especially for him.

tivity." As shall be seen, Henry was only too conscious of all this.

Other mathematical and scientific publications of this early period include works on Fermat[22] and on the theory of numbers,[23] and a publication of new documents on the seventeenth-century Italian scientists Galileo, Torricelli, Cavalieri, and Castelli, also in 1880.[24] Also in 1880, among these scientific and mathematical publications so obviously essential to the development of his system, Henry came out with his first publication relating to the arts, the memoirs of Cochin.[25] Naturally—or significantly—enough, Henry's first publication on art pertains to the classic academic art of the eighteenth century, the "rational" humanistic art developed as a counterpart to rational and objective Cartesian science. Obviously, in order to gain a proper understanding of the total Cartesian world view, Henry found it necessary to take into account the role and function of art, particularly since one of the postulates of modern thought is that somehow science and art are opposed, or at best complement one another. Certainly the academic idea of art maintained in the

22. *Recherches sur les manuscrits de Fermat* (Rome, 1879–80). With Charles Tannery, Henry also edited the monumental *Oeuvres de Fermat,* in four volumes from 1891 to 1912, with a supplement published in 1922. Fermat (1601–65), after Descartes, is certainly the greatest French mathematician of the seventeenth century. Although he rarely published, credit is given to Fermat for the creation of differential calculus and, along with Pascal, the calculus of probabilities. In fact, Fermat had a lively correspondence with Pascal. Most pertinent for Henry's own work is that Fermat was able to represent curves by equations. The *Cercle chromatique,* in a very basic sense, is the reduction of the natural functions to the laws of the circle, different functions being different curves represented by mathematical equations.

23. *Sur divers points de la théorie des nombres* (Paris: Association française pour l'avancement des sciences, 1880).

24. *Galileo, Torricelli, Cavalieri, Castelli, documents nouveaux* (Rome, 1880). The research of the great seventeenth-century scientists was almost always interconnected in one way or another. Thus, Pascal, Torricelli, and Galileo all worked on the barometer and the mercury thermometer.

25. *Mémoires inédites de Charles-Nicolas Cochin sur le comte de Caylus, Bouchardon, et les Slodtz* (Paris: Charavay, 1880).

eighteenth and nineteenth centuries, holding that art and science reigned over two separate realms, those of beauty and knowledge, an idea manifest in the academies established in the seventeenth century, was in need of serious reconsideration. Given what is known of Henry's basic world view, and given the situation with regard to art in his day, it is no surprise that he came to acquire a certain degree of historical knowledge of art in order to have sufficient understanding to create his scientific aesthetic.

The mathematical publications of the early 1880s are increasingly erudite and broadly historical. Among them are works on rapid division,[26] the harmonic triangle,[27] the bibliography of Gergonne,[28] a manuscript of Mydorge's,[29] the works of Gomes de Souza,[30] algorism and geometry,[31] the correspondence of Condorcet and Turgot,[32] Casanova's mathematical knowledge,[33] the geometry of Mydorge,[34] and a mathematical treatise of Condorcet's.[35] What is one to make of all this? First of all, that Henry, who became a librarian at the

26. "Sur un procédé de division rapide," *Nouvelles annales de mathématiques* (1881).

27. *Étude sur le triangle harmonique* (Paris: Gauthier-Villars, 1881).

28. *Supplément à la bibliographie de Gergonne* (Rome, 1882).

29. *Notice sur un manuscrit inédit de Mydorge* (Rome, 1882). Claude Mydorge (1585–1647) studied the properties of light, vision, and refraction, was a close friend of Descartes, and mediated between Descartes and Fermat.

30. *Mémoires de calcul intégral de Joachim Gomes de Souza, publiées avec additions et notices* (Leipzig, 1882). Gomes de Souza was a Brazilian mathematician.

31. *Les deux plus anciens traités français d'algorisme et de géométrie, publiées pour la première fois* (Rome-Paris: Gauthiers-Villars, 1882).

32. *Correspondance inédite de Condorcet et de Turgot* (Paris: Charavay, 1883), Condorcet and Turgot, of course, were two of the leading Enlightenment *philosophes*.

33. *Les connaissances mathématiques de Jacques Casanova de Seingalt* (Rome, 1883).

34. *Problèmes de géométrie pratique de Mydorge*. Enoncés et solutions *publiées* avec commentaires orientaux de M. Leon Rodet (Rome, 1884).

35. *Sur les methodes d'approximation pour les equations differentielles, memoire inédit de Condorcet,* publié avec notice sur les écrits mathématiques (Rome-Paris, 1884).

Chapter Three

Sorbonne in 1881 and held the position until 1892, certainly made use of his post, or fitted himself for it. It is at this time that he became known to his literary and artistic friends Gustave Kahn, Jules Laforgue, and Charles Cros as "le savant." Indeed there is something of the fantastic to Henry's output and breadth of research which truly begins to make itself apparent during this period. The tall, lean Alsatian with blond hair and pale, mountain-lake blue eyes,[36] who has the air of a Doctor Faust and who as a young man rode from Paris to Brussels on a bicycle,[37] commences to take on the role of Faustroll at this point in history.

There is also something in the diverse bibliographical spread of Henry's endeavors that suggests one of those superb tales of Jorge Luis Borges, in which, with just a mere sprinkling of curious names and even more curious titles from as many different historical situations, an entirely new system is hinted at, as in "The Dream of Coleridge" in Borges' *Other Inquisitions*.[38] It is hard to imagine Henry as a youth

36. The description is Gustave Kahn's, in "Hommage à Henry," p. 57.

37. This anecdote comes from Fernand Divoire, "Hommage à Henry," p. 34. There is no reason to doubt this, since Henry was an inordinate bicycle enthusiast. In fact, Henry's interest and activity in bicycling led him to various experiments with the drug Kola and with some synthetic derivatives of this drug with regard to fatigue and stimulation. In these experiments, Henry corresponded with the sociologist Gustave Le Bon. See Henry, "Quelques détails techniques à propos du cyclisme," *Revue blanche* (1894–95) 6:561–67; 7:273–78, 364–68, 459–63, 554–61; 8:235–39, 368–71. In this curious and fantastic series of articles, Henry, already so intellectually stimulated and involved in the concept of circles and cycles, from his own experience develops the mathematical psychophysiology of bicycling!

38. New York, 1965, pp. 13–17. With regard to bibliographical fantasies, another story by Borges is also suggestive of the scholarship of Henry, "Tlön, Uqbar, Orbis Tertius," in *Labyrinths* (New York, 1962) pp. 3–18. In fact, in 1885 Henry published *Pierre de Carcavy*, the papers and biographical note on a librarian and bibliographer of the seventeenth century. In addition to work with Pascal, Roberval, and Fermat, and correspondence with Descartes and Torricelli and Huygens (all men whom Henry had researched or studied), Carcavy was the cataloguer to the royal library and a calligrapher of great repute. Born around 1600, Carcavy, in many ways Henry's seventeenth-century counterpart, died in 1684.

Henry, or Doctor Faustroll

never having any idea of what or whom he was going to be; instead he is one of those who appears full-blown from the forehead of Divine Wisdom and who, from the first, continues to carry out the task at hand as if he had known and remembered it from a previous existence. Kahn writes of Henry at this time: "He took tranquilly the free and difficult way. He was at the same time indecisive and resolute—indecisive solely on deciding which path to follow; fearing failure, he took them all."[39] And indeed this *savant érudit* "with the air of a German student from the Romantic period,"[40] pursued the law of his existence with an uncanny sense of assurance. As his work develops, one observes the way in which his labors reflect the assimilated whole of his endeavors, and one begins to understand that for a man like Henry research is a memory process of a very refined selectivity to be put to use in the creation or, rather, the further creation of a continually self-transforming system. This system can be viewed as the continuing development underlying the principles governing the evolution of consciousness. Henry was indeed the instrument of his labors.

After this early period, Henry's mathematical publications tend to become "mixed" and/or applied to specific problems such as art and aesthetics,[41] or to problems of a more psychophysiological nature such as the measurement of intellectual capacity,[42] the laws governing small numbers,[43] psy-

39. Gustave Kahn, "Hommage à Henry," p. 57.
40. Leouzon le Duc, "Hommage à Henry," p. 61.
41. The most important aesthetic works of the later 1880s and early 1890s are: *Notice sur le rapporteur esthétique* (Paris, 1888); *Cercle chromatique* (1888); *Harmonies de formes et de couleurs* (Paris, 1891); "L'esthétique des formes," *Revue blanche* (1894–95) 7:118–29, 308–22, 511–25; 8:116–20. We will study the chief ideas in these works in chapters 6 and 7 below.
42. *Mesure des capacités intellectuelles et énergétiques* (Paris, 1906).
43. *La loi des petits nombres . . .* (Paris, 1908). Application of the calculus of probabilities, and of Henry's earlier research on the mathematics of Fermat and Pascal.

chobiology and energetics, and others.[44] These publications continue to demonstrate Henry's mathematical versatility and curiosity. Henry's mathematical understanding of phenomena or, rather, his understanding that underlying all phenomena are relationships which can be expressed mathematically, is of such an all-comprehensive nature that it is not surprising that some of the writers compare Henry's effort to that of Pythagoras, and that Henry himself often invokes the name of Pythagoras. Thus George Bohn, writing of Henry's mathematical achievements, states: "It has been said of Charles Henry that he renewed Pythagoras, for, like the latter, he sought to represent the properties of bodies with whole numbers."[45] This connection between Henry and Pythagoras is also another clue, suggesting that Henry belongs as much to the stream of hermetic thought as to the empirical stream. There is to the whole of Henry's life as well as to the nature

44. *Psychobiologie et énergétique: essai sur un principe de méthodes intuitives de calcul* (Paris, 1908). For Henry's doctorate, *Sensation et énergie* and *Mémoire et habitude,* see above, chapter 2, n. 2. Henry's bibliography after the mid 1890s tends to become sketchy. In 1897 there is *Les rayons Röntgens* (Paris: Société des éditions scientifiques). As I have noted already, Henry must be considered one of the pioneers in radiation and x-rays. Röntgen announced his discovery only in 1895. Early in the 1890s Henry was doing research on phosphorescent sulfer of zinc which was then used in industry for the coating of pins and small objects so that they would glow in the dark. From this time on, Henry was intensely involved in the study of radiation. From 1897 to 1906 we know of no publications by Henry, and hence we know very little of him during these years. However, from 1906 to his death twenty years later Henry published again with some regularity, though it is not clear to what extent. There is a bibliography appended to the "Hommage à Henry," but this is most incomplete. The best bibliography of Henry's early works—up to 1888—is given as an appendix to Henry's often bizarre and always informative *Voyages de Balthasar de Monconys,* dedicated to Jules Laforgue and published in 1887. This appendix lists the "principales publications de M. Charles Henry," which number, not including the *Voyages,* thirty-seven books, articles, and so on. Henry was twenty-eight years old in 1887. The *Voyages,* incidentally, makes fascinating reading, containing as it does many detailed accounts of inventions, marvels, curiosities half-scientific and half-occult, much in the manner of the *Natural Magic* of G. Della Porta that was so popular in the late sixteenth and seventeenth centuries.

45. Bohn, "Hommage à Henry," p. 74.

of the ideas developed by him indications of connections which can only be called hermetic. And finally, Henry's mathematics, though having so many historical connections, is, in its *emphasis on simple numbers*, 1, 2, 3, 4, . . . , and their combinations, anticipatory of Planck's quantum theory in which the passage of energy from one element to another is made by 1, 2, 3, 4, . . . , in series of successive bonds or relationships.[46]

Clearly it is not my place to do anything more than suggest Henry's profound involvement in mathematics not as a pure science but as a language or medium by means of which precise translations are made of the various laws governing phenomena, including the very sensations by which it is realized that there are "external phenomena." Certainly it was one of Henry's most successful mathematical endeavors to apply his knowledge to the examination of aesthetic sensations, an endeavor that brought him in direct contact with artists in what can be considered as the first really conscientious effort since Leonardo Da Vinci[47] and the Renaissance to effect a system of vision, or visual and sensorial understanding, that was the product of a blending of the two "separated" realms of beauty and knowledge, art and science. Investigating further this entry of Henry into the art world of the 1880s, it is important to keep in perspective Henry's interest in this matter: it is the interest of a man intent on bringing forth a system which takes into account the totality of human actions, knowledge, and consciousness. In such a system art, as it is commonly understood, is not an autonomous social function nor is it the proof of some doctrine developed in the philosophical subbranch of aesthetics; rather, can art be defined in terms of the extent to which it is a logical function or out-

46. Ibid., pp. 73–74.
47. Indeed, Henry participated in the publication of manuscripts of Leonardo da Vinci by the library of the Institute of France; "Les manuscrits de Léonard de Vinci: manuscrits A et B," *Revue de l'enseignement secondaire et supérieure* (January, 1885).

growth of the sense organ or organs to which it is intended to appeal. In this way art becomes placed again in relation to the natural functions of the senses and of the psychic reactions which attend every physical stimulus. This is the very essence of the psychophysical aesthetic.

Henry's aesthetic is a direct outgrowth of the following idea: "As far as the psychic is to be considered a direct function of the physical, the physical can be called the carrier, the factor underlying the psychical. Physical processes that accompany or underlie psychical functions, and consequently stand in direct functional relationship to them, we shall call psychophysical."[48] One writer describes Henry's *Cercle chromatique* as the work which brought psychophysics out of its embryonic state and transformed it into a rational science, "permitting the rediscovery, through a logical and mathematical way, of the phenomena corresponding to our sensations, of making more precise the laws of our representations of these phenomena, and of producing new states of consciousness."[49] It is worthwhile, then, to try to see how, between the years 1880 and 1884, Henry arrived at his psychophysical aesthetic.

In his introduction to the *Correspondance de Condorcet*, published in 1882, Henry develops in a few pages a sweeping yet thorough understanding of the culture of eighteenth-century France. For this we have to thank Henry the indefatigable librarian, who, in the manner of the librarian of Borges' stories, demonstrates in one article how Descartes' theorem on coordinates stems from the Etruscan numerical notation for 5 (V), and in introducing this edition of Condorcet's correspondence displays a dazzling understanding of the state of knowledge at a given historical moment. In addition to noting the development of ideas leading to the electric telegraph (1774) and the steamboat (1775), as well as to the birth of

48. Fechner, *Elements of Psychophysics,* p. 9.
49. E. Caslant, "Hommage à Henry," p. 97.

socialism, Henry is extraordinarily aware of the situation of the arts in the eighteenth century:

> Art models itself on literature: the aesthetic of Diderot has its artist in Greuze: the pastorals of Gessner are translated in the landscapes of Huet. And there is through the allegories of Lagrenée, the marines of Vernet, the battle scenes of Casanova,[50] the interiors of Chardin, the ruins of Robert, a movement towards the grave: Fragonard, the painter of the *Amours* and the *Graces,* the cherished artist of Madame du Barry and Madame du Pompadour, makes the portrait of Ben Franklin.[51] There is a serious preoccupation with true Antiquity: Vien applies the encaustic which Caylus believes to have rediscovered. . . .[52]

Henry writes with an eye for the significant and a feeling for the seeds of the present. As has been indicated, his eighteenth-century cultural studies began at least as early as 1880 with the publication of the memoirs of Cochin. With special regard to the great dilettante Caylus, Henry, with Henry Cros, published a study in 1884 on the technique of encaustic,[53]

---

50. It should be recalled that the Casanova family was most notable, producing, in addition to two competent painters, the most famous Casanova of them all, Jacques, the famed adventurer, alchemist, diplomat, and mathematician. Needless to say, Henry too fell under the Casanova spell, publishing as he did the mathematical works of Casanova; see above, n. 31.

51. In a later publication by Henry, *Oeuvres et correspondances inédites de d'Alembert* (Paris, 1887), pp. 57–58, Henry reproduces a translation from the Latin of a four-line stanza dedicated to the portrait of Franklin.

52. *Correspondance de Condorcet et de Turgot,* p. x.

53. Charles Henry and Henry Cros, *L'Encaustique et les autres procédés de peinture chez les anciens* (Paris, 1884). Henry Cros was the brother of the litterateur, painter, and experimenter in early color photography, Charles Cros. Henry Cros was a sculptor, and there is evidence that Charles Henry also experimented in sculpture around this time (see below, chapter 4). The Cros brothers were part of the circle which included Kahn and Laforgue, and it was probably through Kahn that Henry met the brothers. It seems altogether possible that Henry Cros' color photography experiments might have been an influence on the neo-impressionist technique of colored dots developed by Seurat and Signac, who might easily have known of the work of Cros, either directly or through Kahn or Henry.

obviously stimulated by the Comte de Caylus' supposed rediscovery of this technique and of his transmitting it to Vien,
the teacher of David; furthermore, in 1886, Henry published
a life of Watteau by the Comte de Caylus, unnoticed by the
Goncourts.[54]

Just as Henry developed a thorough understanding of the
forces at work within and about René Descartes in order to
form a basic working idea of the modern scientific method
and approach, that is, its mathematical basis, in order to better refute and transcend it, so Henry immersed himself in
eighteenth-century studies—but to what end? Though these
studies tend to deal with science and mathematics, there is a
tremendous emphasis on aesthetic values. Although he edited the mathematical works of Condorcet[55] and the correspondence of D'Alembert,[56] Henry's historical interest in the
eighteenth century is broadly cultural. Thus there are his
works on the letters of Mademoiselle Lespinasse,[57] the further correspondence of d'Alembert,[58] the musical theories of
Rameau,[59] Voltaire and Cardinal Quirini,[60] and finally the

54. Charles Henry, *Vie d'Antoine Watteau,* publiée pour la première
fois d'après le manuscrit autographe de M. de Caylus (Paris, 1887).

55. See above, n. 33.

56. Charles Henry, *Correspondance inédite de d'Alembert avec Cramer,
Lesage, Clairaut, Turgot, Castillon, Beguelin . . . ,* D'une notice sur ses travaux mathématiques (Rome-Paris, 1886).

57. *Lettres inédites de Mademoiselle Lespinasse,* avec une étude et
documents nouveaux (Paris, 1887).

58. See above, n. 51.

59. *La théorie de Rameau sur la musique* (Paris, 1887). In the "opus-
cules philosophiques" published in *Oeuvres et correspondance inédites
de d'Alembert* and edited by Henry (Paris, 1887), the *philosophe* writes at
length on the theory of music, generally taking a stand opposed to that
of Rameau. D'Alembert's criticism of Rameau is that the latter, in pursuing
music as an almost purely metaphysical phenomenon, runs the grave risk
of ignoring the laws of nature pertaining to sound as well as the sensation
of sound (pp. 131–89). Henry obviously heeds d'Alembert's criticism,
though not neglecting the virtues of Rameau in formulating the psychophysical theory of music in the *Cercle chromatique.* Indeed, in his Introduction to the *Oeuvres* of d'Alembert, Henry writes, "thus the profound
geometrician was led to study and explain the sentiments of the dilettante.

anonymously published *La vérité sur le Marquis de Sade,* which dates from the same year. Henry's opening observations on the notorious Marquis are not without interest and give a clue to Henry's immersion in eighteenth-century studies: "Sadism will live as long as there is no aesthetic in our lives nor solidarity in our social situation."[61] Though Henry distinguished himself as the ideal private scholar-historian-scientist, he was by no means unaware of the contemporary situation, and one senses that his observation on the Marquis de Sade is totally applicable to the 1880s, which had their own "decadents." Certainly, there was no one unifying aesthetic in Henry's day, as there is not in ours, much less social solidarity. Given his broad studies in the history of science, French culture, and mathematics, Henry must also have been aware that the Cartesian world view had inadequately accounted for the "subjective" aspect of existence, that as-

---

D'Alembert had full consciousness of the importance of a scientific aesthetic" (p. xiii). Thus Henry quotes d'Alembert: "In discovering the true sources of this pleasure [of harmony in music] we would be able to find therein the means of procuring for us in this genre new pleasures. We would then make music like the construction of eye-glasses, which have received such great degrees of perfection since the discovery of the true laws of refraction and light." Indeed, this is but another historical cue for the construction of Henry's chromatic circle, the exposition of his own scientific aesthetic.

60. *Voltaire et le cardinal Quirini* (Paris: Dentu, 1887). Also by Henry, from the same publisher in the same year, was the *Introduction à la chymie, manuscrit inédit de Denis Diderot.* With regard to this last text, which, incidentally, we were unable to locate, we did find a reference to it in the *Manuel bibliographique des sciences psychiques ou occultes,* (Paris, 1912) 2:251 in which Albert C. Caillet comments that the introduction to the chemistry of Diderot by Henry contains a curious theory about the ancient alchemists Bacon, Paracelsus, von Helmont, Zozymus, Basil Valentinus, Albertus Magnus, and others. Whatever this theory is, here again we find evidence that Henry was acquainted to a greater or lesser degree with not only the history of modern science, as we call it, but with the history of the traditional sciences, including alchemy, as well. *Voltaire and Cardinal Quirini,* by the way, was dedicated to Félix Fénéon.

61. Quoted in J-F Revel, "Charles Henry," p. 58. Henry's work on the Marquis de Sade was apparently published anonymously by Dentu, the publisher of Henry's works on Voltaire, Diderot, and Watteau.

pect which is popularly given over to the feelings and to art. Left unchecked, the subjective aspect of existence undergoes hypertrophy and results in such exotic emotional flowers as envisioned by the diabolical Marquis, the final product of the Age of Enlightenment. In fact, the entire phenomenon of Romanticism can be seen as kind of a Cartesian "revenge" principle: initial emphasis upon and overdevelopment of the objective, "rational," intellectual, and scientific, at the expense and, in a basic sense, neglect of the emotional, intuitive, "irrational" aspect of being. This emphasis leads to ultimate emotional excesses, misunderstandings, and outbreaks that finally threaten the entire structure.

Basing himself on the total culture of Descartes—the Cartesian knowledge system—Henry sought to correct the errors growing out of it: sadism, romanticism, unenlightened indulgence in and exploitation of emotion—the sentimentality which can certainly be said to be the aesthetic opiate of the masses, in Henry's time as well as today. In the early 1880s Henry began to devise his scientific aesthetic in order to bring into line the two factors separated by the Cartesian dualistic assumption. The first step that has been indicated was historical research in order to have a clear *causal* grasp of the situation: it is to this end that Henry published research on the art and culture of the prime Cartesian epoch, the Age of Enlightenment, as well as on some manuscripts by, significantly enough, the arch artist-scientist, Leonardo da Vinci. Having a grasp of the historical roots of the contemporary aesthetic dilemma, Henry took a second step involving two aspects: familiarity with contemporary science—a relatively scholarly and intellectual task or form of research—and familiarity with the contemporary cultural situation. One cannot ascertain how consciously Henry set himself to this task, and how much of it may have been due to "chance"; perhaps, and most likely, it was the result of both, as certain circumstances in his involvement in the cultural life of the 1880s seem to indicate. Concerning the first aspect of the second step, knowledge of contemporary scientific developments, it need only be said for the moment that this came "naturally" to the mathematically inclined Henry, but that, even so, his capacity to keep up with the changes in science had something of the extraordinary about it. Indeed, Henry's scientific, that is, psychophysical, experimentation in the 1880s is inseparable from his aesthetic. This in turn was most influential on the arts of the period—certainly the visual arts and literature were directly affected by his research. It is more difficult to determine the effect of Henry's work on music, not that he neglected the study of musical sensation.

Henry's musical studies include those on musical sensation,[62] Rameau,[63] and Wronski,[64] all published in 1886–87. These studies show a threefold interest on the part of Henry which is part and parcel of his general aesthetic:

1. A mathematical interest that is Pythagorean in origin; this should not be at all surprising considering Henry's Pythagorean and even Platonic attitude to the function of music in the regulation of life. Rameau and Wronski can also be related to the Pythagorean approach in terms of the mysticism of number.
2. An interest in the evolution of a given sense function.
3. A concern with the nature of the auditory/musical sense itself, that is, the psychophysical consideration, whose mathematical approach completes the circuit of Henry's method.

Henry's musical ideas, in addition to forming an integral part of his universal aesthetic, also are in line with the demands of the time best revealed by the Wagnerian dictum of the

62. Charles Henry, "Loi d'évolution de la sensation musicale," *Revue philosophique* 22:81–87.
63. See above, n. 59.
64. *Wronski et l'esthétique musicale* (Paris, 1887). With regard to a mathematical transcendental aesthetic, Wronski is one of Henry's chief sources, although next to nothing is known about this nineteenth-century Polish scientist.

gesamkunstwerke, the synesthetic experience. Furthermore, Henry's approach to music as an aspect of the unfolding of consciousness, as well as his understanding of music—harmony and rhythm—as a fundamental life function, is unique in itself, though not without historical basis.[65] Finally, verifying Kahn's contention that the symbolic, transcendental theory of art could be traced to Henry,[66] we need only quote again: "Musica est excercitum arithemeticae occultae nescentis se numerare animi."

One can begin to glimpse the development of the intellectual structure of the universal system envisioned by Charles Henry. Basing himself on the universal language of mathematics, Henry applied this language in two ways: as a Cartesian instrument of precise measurement, and as a Pythagorean language of symbols. With an acute awareness of universal complementarities and the dualism which can be engendered if the universal polarities are not properly understood, Henry meant to effect the union of opposites, an aim which, when applied to the culture of his time, was to be first expressed as the creation of a scientific aesthetic. But more than intellect and observation is necessary to create an idea: experience and spirit must also be utilized, or as Santayana writes:

> It is not wisdom to be only wise
> and on inner vision close the eyes—
> but it is wisdom to follow the heart.

65. An interesting present-day follow-up to Henry's musical ideas is Alain Danielou, "The Influence of Sound on Consciousness," *Psychedelic Review,* no. 7 (1966):20–26. Like Henry in the *Cercle Chromatique,* Danielou applies the psychophysiological analysis of sound to language as well. Indeed the theory of the *mantras,* the sacred sounds and syllables of the Tantric traditions, is a pure manifestation of the idea of linguistic sound used specifically as an agent acting upon the states of consciousness, with the intention of altering or expanding consciousness. Rimbaud's concept of the vowels is related to the mantric function of sound.

66. In his "Réponse des symbolistes," of 1886 (see above, chapter 1, n. 5) Kahn makes this pronouncement, indicating as well that Henry was a "philosophe esoterique."

Henry, or Doctor Faustroll

For this reason it is well to turn to a study, if it may be called that, of the disposition of Henry's "heart" in the early 1880s.

4

Charles Henry, the Guardian Angel of Laforgue's Complaints

HENRY the erudite, the genius savant, moves across these pages like a shadow, a bibliography in search of a personality. What is known of Henry as a person in the 1880s? What was the nature of his interpersonal relationships with poets and painters alike? Little is known about this factor, and obviously it is more difficult to determine the exact nature of these relationships. Long before Henry became involved with the painters of the neo-impressionist movement, he formed very significant relationships with a number of writers and certainly came into intimate contact with contemporary cultural figures. Perhaps the most important of these friendships was that which Henry sustained for the duration of the brief career of the brilliant poet and litterateur Jules Laforgue.[1]

Though this is no place for a thorough study of the relationship between Henry and Laforgue—to the best of my knowledge no such study has yet been undertaken, though

---

1. Perhaps still the best account of Laforgue's life is the study by François Ruchon (see above, chapter 1, n. 11). A fair English account is Michael Collie, *Laforgue* (Edinburgh, 1963). See also, William J. Smith, *Selected Writings of Jules Laforgue* (New York, 1956). Of the complete works of Laforgue edited by G. Jean-Aubry we have had recourse in particular to the volumes of letters (*Oeuvres complètes,* vols. 4, 5 [Paris, 1922]).

The Guardian Angel

it would certainly be worthwhile[2]—it is more than obvious that much of Laforgue's thought and approach bears the hallmark of Henry's studies. Laforgue's writings on the impressionist painters are certainly much in debt to ideas similar to those generated by Henry. Though little is known of Henry's youth, there is much that can be gleaned from that of Laforgue, whom Henry met, probably in 1879, through another close literary acquaintance, Gustave Kahn.[3] In 1879, Henry had been in Paris for some four years and was living on the Rue Berthollet, the same street where the young Laforgue lived, who was then acting out the "sufferings" of a young poet. "I was once a tragic Buddhist," Laforgue wrote in 1882, "and now I am a dilettante Buddhist."[4] To what extent Henry participated in the young poet's religious crisis at this early period is unclear. There is in Henry's writings no indication of a crisis on his part, and in fact Henry seems to have set himself on an even keel on religious matters quite early in his career. This does not at all mean that Henry did not con-

2. One such study has been made. See Georges Pillement, "Charles Henry et Jules Laforgue," in "Hommage à Henry," pp. 66–70. Pillement's description of Henry is not without interest: "When I knew Charles Henry, he was already an old man, a great old man, astonishingly thin, ataxic, supporting himself on your arm to cross the street. But he had, despite his age and illness, something extraordinarily young in his clear eyes which recalled the bohemian of his adolescence, and which appeared to me of great prestige: he had been the friend of Jules Laforgue, and he had not become an official scholar, stiff and vain; he had remained independent, a little bit bohemian, he had something Laforguean about him" (p. 66). On the other hand, Pillement's account is not particularly revealing of the relationship between Laforgue and Henry.

3. Kahn writes of knowing Henry in 1879, and recalls seeing him on the rue Mazarine, leaving the Bibliothèque de l'Institut, dressed—at nineteen years of age—in black and wearing a top hat, which Kahn states was something of a uniform for Henry ("Hommage à Henry," p. 57). Actually, it is really not clear precisely how the three came together; all that is known is that sometime in 1879–80, perhaps at one of the libraries, Kahn, Laforgue, and Henry slowly came into one another's acquaintance, a mutual acquaintance that was fateful for all concerned. Kahn and Laforgue met first at the Club des hydropaths.

4. Quoted in Smith, *Writings of Laforgue*, p. 6.

cern himself about religion. In 1878, after all, he published Bossuet's treatise on the knowledge of God,[5] and, as has been already noted, toward the end of his life, Henry publicly acknowledged that the theory he had finally worked out had in many ways been better achieved or known by those who had created other systems, namely Buddha and Pythagoras. Almost from the start Henry's career seems possessed of a singular clarity of purpose marked out by his works along the way; from the beginnings under the discipleship of Claude Bernard, the experimental doctor, to the final summation of the theory of radiation, Henry's life exhibits a singular case of "path-consciousness,"[6] to use Lama Govinda's words. Thus, although it is the young Laforgue who manifests the spiritual malaise of the century of Baudelaire, it is Henry who guides to spiritual clarity under the guise of positivist science. An indication of this is seen in a letter from Laforgue to Henry written in April of 1882, shortly after Laforgue had begun his curious role as reader to the German court:[7]

5. See above, chapter 3, n. 10. Collie, *Laforgue,* p. 13 writes, "Kahn also introduced Laforgue to another unreligious intellectual, Charles Henry." To us this is a most shortsighted assessment.

6. Govinda, *Early Buddhist Philosophy,* p. 101: "In the supramundane consciousness which, by the way, is tied to no definite plane or form of consciousness, but may dwell in all domains, the active aspect [of Karma, the law of ethical retribution which includes the concept of reincarnation] is designated as Path-consciousness." In the case of Henry himself, for whom the matter of afterlife—*survie*—was both a matter of faith and scientific proof, it is clear that he suggests something of a conscious and willed continuity from life to life. As fantastic as they may seem, here and there one does come across such bizarre figures as the eighteenth-century Comte de St.-Germain who boasted that he "lived forever." Such a phrase may be a metaphor for the conscious and willed continuity through a succession of lives; thus the "work" of each life picks up where the last left off. It is also interesting that some of Henry's very last publications deal with the specific theme of postmortem survival.

7. Recommended by Charles Ephrussi, then editor of the *Gazette des beaux-arts,* and Paul Bourget, Laforgue obtained in 1881 the position of French reader to the German court, a job that plunged Laforgue into what can best be called a state of creative spleen.

The Guardian Angel

My dear friend Henry,

How you must have it in for me! But if you only knew into what a state of despair I have sunk—deeper and deeper. . . . I received your most "eloquent" letter just as I was leaving Berlin. I wanted to formulate a suitable reply to the advice you gave me, but I have hardly unpacked my trunks. . . . I am bored, that's all that's to it. I feel the emptiness of everything, love, glory, art, metaphysics.

There are some days when one cheerfully tells oneself that universal life is only a transitory kaleidoscope —and other days when, were it not for the retina of the human brain, this kaleidoscope would consist of nothing but vibrations. But on other days, that's where I am.

I am hardly writing at all, but I think a great deal— and I am indeed convinced that I am not just scraping a literary guitar.

You who have gone through Spinoza and Berkeley,[8] who have gone to the depths of human thought, what do you say about that? Have you been through this crisis of spleen? I can hear you asking me what the trouble is. I'm not anemic anymore. I haven't got heart trouble anymore. I haven't got a thing to worry about. I have nothing to do. I breathe an air which never circulated in the Bibliotheque nationale. I want nothing, nothing whatever. . . .

8. An indication that Henry, whose thought was characterized by Mirabaud as "scientific idealism," was early imbued with classic idealist philosophy. For instance, in the Third Dialogue of *Hylas and Philonous,* first published by Berkeley in 1713, Hylas replies: "Words are not to be used without a meaning. And, as there is no more meaning in *spiritual Substance* than in *material Substance,* the one is to be exploded as well as the other" (Berkeley, *Three Dialogues Between Hylas and Philonous* [Chicago, 1959], p. 95). Some two hundred years later Henry wrote, towards the conclusion of his *Généralisation de la théorie du rayonnement:* "The old metaphysical idea of 'substance,' in creating in the spirit of many specialists an abyss between the so-called domain of thought and that of matter, has been one of the most fatal ideas to the progress of Science" (p. 139).

Chapter Four

I long to see you. Do you want me to send you some poems?

I wanted to write to Kahn. You gave me his address, I believe, but I shan't be able to locate your letter before settling down in Baden-Baden.

I have been designing a funeral bed that I shall have built when I have an apartment in Paris. . . .[9]

It is clear from this letter that Henry, although only one year Laforgue's senior, is playing a role much closer to that of teacher than intellectual peer. Laforgue treats Henry as if he were a person of much greater experience, or at least experience of a different order, and it would appear that this was at the core of the relationship. Indeed this can be discerned at the earliest point of the relationship between the two young men. François Ruchon describes how Laforgue came into contact with another curious member of the literati, the mysterious Sandah Mahali (Mlle Multzer). "Sandah Mahali, whom he (Laforgue) knew through M. Charles Henry, was a likeable woman, friend of the arts, kind of a poet herself in her more intimate moments, and who held a salon on the Rue Denfort-Rochereau: 'This intimate and dark salon with the severe furnishings,' received every Sunday at nightfall, poets, musicians, men of letters."[10]

It can be established that certainly by 1879–80 Henry was already making his way through the literary demimonde of Paris, while pursuing at the same time his research in the investigation and history of certain fundamental psychophysical problems. Laforgue at this time was attending Taine's

9. Laforgue, *Oeuvres* 4:144–46, Letter 34 (April 22, 1882). Altogether, Laforgue addressed fifty-eight letters to Henry between 1881 and 1886. This particular letter is also reproduced in Smith, *Writings of Laforgue*, pp. 244–45.

10. Ruchon, *Jules Laforgue*, p. 24. Very little is known of Mme Mahali, actually Mlle Multzer, the estranged wife of a Parisian architect, some thirteen years the senior of Laforgue and Henry. Indeed how Henry came into contact with this woman is totally unclear, but it is curious that it is the "scientist" who made the initial introduction.

The Guardian Angel

lectures on art at the Sorbonne and immersing himself in Schopenhauer, Buddhism, Darwin, and Hartmann's philosophy of the unconscious.[11] Later, Laforgue was to write most affectionately to Henry of these early days, so much in evidence in the letter already quoted: "Where are our evenings on the rue Seiguier and rue Berthollet, our walks along the rue de l'Abée de l'Epée, to the Boulevard Port Royal, and past the carnival of the avenue des Gobelins with our singular conversations?"[12] Certainly Henry was sympathetic to the young poet, and while Laforgue was working out his "Buddhist" phase with its pronounced emphasis on asceticism, Henry was the person with whom Laforgue was in closest contact. No doubt Henry functioned as Laforgue's scientific and philosophical mentor, as well as personal guide, friend,

11. Eduard von Hartmann, 1842–1906. According to Hall, *Modern Psychology*, pp. 238–39, "Hartmann's proof of the eccentric, penumbral, peripheral, marginal nature of consciousness makes him a modern Copernicus. The erection of the Unconscious as a world-principle marks the great revolution of views since the Renaissance, which was its prelude, in emancipating the world from the views of the past. . . . If we ever have a new idealism in the world again, it will be somewhat along the lines of Hartmann's Unconscious.

"Hartmann's chief significance lies in his advocacy of the Unconscious and his opposition to the 'consciousness philosophies,' which had been in vogue ever since Descartes. He saw more clearly than did even Comte (who rejected psychology in his hierarchy of sciences because of the fallacies inherent in introspection) their fallacies. To him, even more than to Lotze or even Fechner, Kant was the arch sophist, the Protagoras of modern times, because he taught distrust of the senses, which alone give us true reality." Hartmann's *Philosophie des Unbewussten* [Philosophy of the unconscious], first published in 1869, was perhaps the most powerful single intellectual influence on Laforgue, and we can infer that it had some influence upon Henry as well. With regard to Henry, this influence is best seen in the idea of a cosmic evolutionary principle in which consciousness is continually transforming itself into ever more expanded states. Thus we can see the basic dynamic sources of the aesthetic of which Laforgue dreamed, an aesthetic representing one law, one universal mystic principle—the same aesthetic which Henry strove to articulate, the aesthetic of transcendental beauty. See also Mederic Dufour, *Etude sur l'esthétique de Jules Laforgue* (Paris, 1904), pp. 20ff. Dufour mentions a very strong influence of Henry's researches on Laforgue, but is never very specific.

12. Laforgue, *Oeuvres*, 4:143, letter 33 (April 16, 1882).

Chapter Four

and confidant. The relationship he established with Laforgue can be taken as the model for Henry's later friendships with the painters Seurat and Signac.

A further image of Henry is contained in the following poem written by Laforgue in a letter to his Parisian friend, on December 5, 1881, and which I translate here:

> My dear Henry,
> An evening went its long steps . . . to the Sorbonne,
>   A corpulent napkin upon its arm,
> Henry! some black street-arabs—they pleased his person,
>   but him—great—they did not see!
> In a hurry, he smiled to the gloom-worn chimneys,
>   hearts of gold in tin-plate tubes,
> and these daughters, mined from a sooty spleen,
>   saluted this noctambulant.[13]

This certainly testifies to a warm, intimate, and most respectful understanding of Henry. The correspondence at this time reveals a lively intellectual relationship as well. Mention is made of Stendhal, of an anthology which Laforgue and Henry planned to make, of Baudelaire, Degas, Manet, Monet, and Forain, Kate Greenaway and Max Klinger. More specifically relating to Henry, in a letter dated January, 1882, Laforgue expresses amazement at Henry's many ventures, including the study of encaustic,[14] the anesthesiometer,[15] Fermat and

13. Ibid., p. 45.

14. Obviously in preparation for the book which Henry published jointly with Henry Cros (see above, chapter 3, n. 53); from what Laforgue has to say in his letters it would seem that Henry did a bit of experimenting in sculpture and painting, undoubtedly in conjunction with Cros. Laforgue, *Oeuvres*, 4:90–93.

15. Mention of the anesthesiometer at this time indicates that as early as January, 1882, Henry was engaged in actual psychophysical experimentation. The anesthesiometer was obviously a device for measuring states of *anesthesia*. It is possible that this is also one of the sources of the scientific aesthetic which Henry developed later in the 1880s: what is an *anaesthetic* state if not the opposite of an *aesthetic* one? In Henry's later psychobiological terminology, anaesthesia is a state of acute *inhibition;* aesthesia, the "aesthetic experience" in traditional terminology, is a state of *dynamogeny.*

60

The Guardian Angel

Caylus. Then there is the testimony of a certain journalist, Lindenlaub,[16] who comments to Laforgue on Henry's "singularity" as a person, whereas Sandah Mahali writes, "yes, Henry is an extraordinary being."[17] In perhaps the most telling incident, Henry has asked Laforgue to get in touch with the ambassador from Brazil in Germany with regard to Henry's publication of the memoirs of Gomes de Souza. When Laforgue finally interceded for Henry, the Brazilian ambassador, Jaurus, who had already been apprised of Henry's publications and interests, expressed to the poet his belief that Henry must be at least forty years old. Henry was then twenty-two. Further testifying to the nature of their relationship is a letter containing a great deal of verse, obviously intended for Henry's critical opinion, in which the poet assures Henry that in a month and a half he will be back in Paris where the two will be able to continue their promenades, "from the cold quais of the Seine to the burning banks of the Ganges."[18] For finally, by Laforgue's own pronouncement, Charles Henry was "constituted the guardian angel of my [Laforgue's] complaints."[19]

Indeed, *aesthetics,* which comes from the Greek word "aisthanesthai," to be sensitive, to perceive, would seem to be one of the necessary domains of the true psychophysicist. Thus, in Henry's doctrine, the most healthy, normal, and dynamogenous states experienced by any organism are inherently aesthetic!

16. Theodore Lindenlaub was a Parisian journalist who apparently knew Henry in Paris, and who became acquainted with Laforgue in Berlin.

17. Laforgue, *Oeuvres,* 4:103, letter to Mme Mullezer (sic) (January 23, 1882). In letters to Mme Multzer as well as to Kahn, there is often mention of Henry.

18. Ibid., p. 166, letter 41 (June 5, 1882).

19. Ibid., 5:84, letter 88 (June, 1884). Also in this letter Laforgue mentions an article by Georges Geroult published in the *Gazette des beaux-arts* (1882):165, entitled "Formes, couleurs, mouvements." This article is certainly one of the sources of the idea that both Laforgue and Henry develop relating the visual sensation to a progressive degradation of light, color, and form with the sense of movement implied in the degradation from the state of pure light to the least pure, or most complicated of form. See also, by the same writer, an article of the preceding year which also must have received attention from Laforgue and Henry, "Du rôle du mouvement des

Chapter Four

What can be gleaned of Henry's own thought from the letters of Laforgue is also not without interest. Obviously he was very philosophically inclined (the mention of Berkeley and Spinoza) and, in addition, had developed a certain equanimity in which Laforgue found some kind of refuge. There is even some hint of what might be considered a metaphysical bent on Henry's part reflected in Laforgue's rhapsodic comment that "universal life is only a transitory kaleidoscope";[20] or, if not that, "were it not for the retina of the *human* brain, this kaleidoscope would consist of nothing but vibrations." In this passage Buddhism and psychophysics glide one into the other. The "transitory kaleidoscope" is a particularly "Buddhist" metaphor; thus the kaleidoscopic Buddhist phrase:

As stars, a fault of vision, as a lamp,
A mock show, dew drops, or a bubble,
so should we view what is conditioned [that is, existence].[21]

And yet, there is the more psychophysical interjection concerning the "retina of the human brain," without which medium the kaleidoscope would "consist of nothing but vi-

---

yeux dans les émotions esthétiques," *Gazette des beaux-arts* 6, pts. 1, 2 (1881):536ff; 7, pt. 1 (1882):82ff. These articles are most significant in view of the theory of directions and interior work that Henry later develops, and certainly indicate a fundamentally psychophysical approach to aesthetic studies.

20. In addition to the mention of the kaleidoscope in the letter I have quoted (see above, n. 9), Laforgue uses this image in corresponding with Henry in a letter dated May 5, 1882 (*Oeuvres*, 4:157). Laforgue writes, "Brief, all the kaleidoscope of life. But one is quite miserable and finished at the base of things when life has only the interest of a kaleidoscope for you, isn't that so?" And in a letter to Henry dated January, 1885 (ibid., 5:106), Laforgue states that he "adores 'Kaleidoscope,'" a poem by Verlaine published in Verlaine's book of verse, *Jadis et naguère*. It is well to keep this image of the kaleidoscope in mind when viewing the *Portrait of Fénéon* by Signac, a work in which Henry's ideas are most apparent and which I shall discuss below in chapter 7.

21. From the Vajrachedikka, quoted in E. Conze, et al., *Buddhist Texts through the Ages* (New York, 1964), p. 161.

brations." This idea transmitted as it probably was from Helmholtz, Hartmann, and Fechner, also has its points of contact with Buddhist psychology. Consider the following verse from the *Lalitavistara*:

> Dependent on eye and sight-object
> An act of eye-consciousness springs up here.
> But the sight-object is not based on the eye,
> Nor has any sight-object been transferred to the eye.[22]

Can Henry have known much if anything about Buddhism at this time? It is difficult to say, although one writer states that Henry was studying Sanskrit in the late 1870s,[23] and several of Henry's articles on the history of mathematics published in 1879 in the *Revue archéologique* contain facts pertaining to the mathematical systems of the various oriental peoples including the Arabs, the Indians, and the Chinese. Most likely, whatever "Buddhist" knowledge Henry and Laforgue possessed between them was gained by a mutually contributory method.

The mention of "vibrations" may be the richest and most suggestive key of all. As shall be seen, Laforgue is the one impressionist critic to make the most use out of the concept of "vibrations," and this is not at all surprising considering his friendship with Henry. The concept of vibrations is one that is innate to psychophysics, since certain sense-phenomena are directly related to the physical phenomenon of the electromagnetic spectrum, which is defined in terms of frequency of vibrations. Of course, vibrations in this sense would have gained impetus at this time due to Clerk Max-

22. Ibid., p. 159. A truly excellent study of the phenomena of vision in which theories much like this one are discussed is Vasco Ronchi, *L'optique: science de vision* (Paris, 1966). Also of the greatest significance is Govinda, *Early Buddhist Philosophy*, pp. 134ff, for the discussion of the processes of perception, as well as for the appendixes to this book, which is really a commentary on the ancient Buddhist text the *Abhidhamma*, the fundamental statement of Buddhist psychophysiology.

23. Doyen, "Hommage à Henry," p. 37.

well's discovery in 1878 of the electromagnetic nature of heat and light—radiation—a discovery to which Henry most certainly attuned himself, as he did in 1897 with his publication on Roentgen's discovery of X-rays (1895), and as he finally did with his *Généralisation de la théorie du rayonnement*. But vibrations are phenomena not related solely to the vocabulary of Western physics, but again to Buddhist thought, as well as to more occult systems. On the other hand, it is not at all surprising that some of the early researchers in electricity and electromagnetic phenomena, such as Maxwell, Sir Oliver Lodge, and even Thomas Alva Edison, later in their careers became concerned with psychic or occult phenomena precisely because of their research into the nature of vibrations. In this respect too, a comparison of Henry with another famous nineteenth-century psychophysicist, Edwin Babbitt is worthwhile. For instance, keeping in mind Laforgue's kaleidoscope metaphor in the letter to Henry, we read in Babbitt's *Principles of Light and Color*, published in 1878: "Several times I have seen untold millions of polarized particles of vari-colored luminous matter, changing their lines of polarity scores of times a second like an infinite kaleidoscope, and yet never falling into disorder, for when a particle left one line it would immediately form in exact order in the next line."[24]

There is one other matter from the Laforgue letter to Henry that is worth taking into consideration, and that is the possibility that Henry in one way or another served as Laforgue's "therapist." Thus when the poet states: "I can hear you ask-

24. Edwin Babbitt, *Principles of Light and Color*, ed. Faber Birren (New Hyde Park, 1967), p. 185. Babbitt, a self-proclaimed psychophysicist, after a serious optical ailment early in the 1870s, developed a totally cosmic principle of light and color that is expressed in language or ideas that are often very similar to Henry's in the *Cercle chromatique,* though Babbitt is exuberant where Henry is reticent or poetically precise. Nevertheless, the two cover much of the same ground. See also Faber Birren, *Color Psychology and Color Therapy* (New Hyde Park, 1961). Birren is an excellent example of a modern psychophysicist much in the manner of Henry or Chevreul.

The Guardian Angel

ing me what the trouble is. I'm not anemic any more. I haven't got heart trouble any more . . . ," there is a suggestion that Henry, who had studied under Claude Bernard, was relied upon to "diagnose" Laforgue's symptoms. If this was indeed the case, most certainly the symptoms must have been proven by Henry to have been entirely psychosomatic.

Further hints emphasizing Henry's character may be gleaned from other letters that Laforgue addressed to Henry as well as to others during the poet's years in Germany. In a letter dated August, 1883, Laforgue asks Henry: "Are you often in? Hardly at all I suppose, except in the evening—neither the circus nor the theatre interest you."[25] So we see Henry the solitary scholar, almost, one is tempted to say, the ascetic that Laforgue himself aspired to be. And in a letter dated July, 1884, Laforgue writes: "It is one o'clock, and I haven't yet washed and dressed. I'll be leaving for Constance in half an hour. In the main I continue to lead the same empty life. It really is time for me to do something else. *You have mapped out a life for yourself and seem happy and whole* while I just go on drifting. [Emphasis added.] I should have been able to save enough money in these three years to leave this place, return to Paris, and loaf for about a year until something turned up. So you see, I live in the bosom of the Unconscious; and the Unconscious will take care of me."[26] Psychologically, this paragraph is most revealing, and more than bears out the intuition of Charles Henry, pursuer of "path-consciousness," who had recognized already in his labors the design of his destiny on a level beyond that of the great unconscious where Laforgue resigned himself. In a curious way it is Henry, the scholar of the *vita contemplativa,* who is in the active function of probing consciousness, whereas the poet with as sure a sense of fate as Henry's remains a receptive function of the unconscious. Though the two men shared much of their lives together during the summer, with

25. Laforgue, *Oeuvres,* 5:44.
26. Ibid., pp. 95–96.

Chapter Four

Laforgue's fiancée Miss Leah Lee, in a little cottage near Chevreuse,[27] they develop a relationship in which Laforgue is the recipient agent—which does not make him any the less creative for it—and Henry is the moving agent—which does not make him less receptive to Laforgue's talents and experience.

For instance, Henry was most helpful to Laforgue with his first published book of verse, *Les complaintes de la vie*. It was to Henry that Laforgue addressed this endeavor in 1883, and it was Henry finally who, through his encouragement and literary connections, saw the *Complaintes* through to its publication in 1885. It would not be too farfetched to state that in one way or another Henry helped with the creation of this important work to the extent that without him Laforgue would never have seen the work to its end. Here we see Henry functioning in a most sensitive and encouraging way, helping to guide a work of art through its creation in much the same way as he must later have seen the works of Seurat and Signac to their completion.

On the other hand, evidence of Henry's own "artistic" bent is to be gleaned from another aspect of the relation between the scientist and the poet—Laforgue's gentle insistence that Henry write a novel. This request on the part of Laforgue appears in a number of letters. For example, the poet asks of Henry in August of 1883:

> What are you doing? All these days passed in Paris you seem to have been vaguely doing nothing. Harness yourself to a novel. Between us, I would wish this with a most singular and a most sincere curiosity. At your age you have an enormous grasp of science, of what is in books and of life; put yourself into a novel; give us some of the riches drawn absolutely from your bottomless depths. For you have dreamed it and all of it is to be put in its place. Moreover you know that this is all

27. See Warren Ramsay, *Jules Laforgue and the Ironic Inheritance* (New York, 1953), p. 39.

there is to the world, and you bear within you the consciousness of being and of the race.[28]

A curious and supreme appraisal of Henry by the young poet. In an earlier letter, Laforgue asks Henry if he is making any wax sculpture with Charles Cros and adds, "When will you decide then to make something for which you are so well prepared, to cast forth a novel that is really new? Above all, you who have never written any verse, but have marched into life dressed up in erudition and mathematics. When?"[29] And a year or so later, Laforgue asks again, "What have you done? I see everywhere signs of your book. Could you send me a copy. In any case my best regards. But when will your novel or poems in prose appear?"[30]

It would seem that Henry had indeed prepared a novel, a prose poem entitled, most appropriately, "Vision," which culminated with a reference to the music of the last scene of Wagner's *Die Meistersinger* and was published in the first issue of *La vogue*.[31] Be that as it may, Henry's literary forays were of a far more scholarly nature. In many ways Henry might appear more the literary or artistic entrepreneur if it were not also for the fact that he, as much as any of the artists and literati, helped to fashion the transcendental aesthetic of the Parisian avant-garde of the 1880s.

But with a man like Henry, what is one to expect? Laforgue indicates that in Henry there was the wealth of knowledge and experience necessary to create a *new* novel. Perhaps in his own way, Henry did as much in the publication of previ-

---

28. Quoted in Pillement, "Hommage à Henry," p. 58, as October, 1882, but in Laforgue, *Oeuvres*, 5:47, letter 76 indicates August 22, 1883; Pillement is obviously in error.

29. Laforgue, *Oeuvres*, 4:200, letter 53 (October 13, 1882).

30. Ibid., 5, letter 71 (July 14, 1883). The book to which Laforgue refers is probably *Correspondance inédite de Condorcet et de Turgot*.

31. For Laforgue's comment when Henry's "Poem en prose" finally appeared see above, chapter 2, n. 22. It is possible that Henry wrote other such pieces which were never published. See Kahn, Pillement, in "Hommage à Henry."

Chapter Four

ously unedited historical material. As has already been observed, these publications are not unrelated units, but form
something of a web whose logic and meaning are to be
grasped only in an understanding of the whole and of the
purpose guiding the evolution of the structure as a whole. Is
this not what is asked of a novel, that its parts be so related
as to create a whole whose meaning is to be found in the
purpose guiding the development of the structure, the organic relationship of the parts? An indication that Henry himself thought of his work in something like this manner is to
be gleaned in a statement that concludes the introduction to
the letters of Mademoiselle Lespinasse, dated October, 1886,
in which Henry discloses his purpose for publishing this
book: "The present volume ought to be considered as the
complement of these three publications: The *Correspondance de Condorcet et Turgot, Oeuvres et Correspondances
inédites de d'Alembert, Correspondance inédite de d'Alembert.*[32] Certainly here Henry has created a web of relationships
between these characters from the eighteenth century that in
many respects has all the fascination and depth of a novel, a
genuinely historical novel, an entertainment created from the
very fabric of what is called history. Just as the earliest nov-
els, which in many ways Mlle Lespinasse reflects in her own
correspondence, were compilations of letters, so Henry's
"novel" consists of compilations of history. In any case, the
"Study of Mlle Lespinasse" written in 1882, some four years
prior to its publication with the *Lettres,* is a warm and even
passionate statement giving the impression that Henry himself was only the latest of the lovers of the eighteenth-century
dame[33] whose charm lay precisely in seducing even the most

32. Henry, *Lettres de Mlle de Lespinasse,* p. 7.
33. Indeed though the *Lettres* were not published until 1887, as early
as 1882 Henry was apparently waxing enthusiastic over Mlle Lespinasse,
for Laforgue, *Oeuvres,* 4:185, letter 48, comments to Henry: "Mlle Lespinasse interests me immensely; are you in love with her?" And in ibid.,
5:14, letter 63 (March, 1883), Laforgue, who has received a copy of the
essay which was to serve as the preface to the letters of Mlle de Lespinasse

68

The Guardian Angel

philosophical of spirits such as Henry's predecessor, D'Alembert. Henry writes:

> Mademoiselle de Lespinasse crossed the threshold of posterity and will live as long as there is passion; she will live at the side of Sappho, of St. Theresa, of Heloise, at the side of those rare ones who have written with strength for having lived strongly. And that is perpetual literature: literatures succeed one another, systems change, tastes pass, fashions whirl about, life remains. . . . She will live as saint and martyr of an immortal religion: Love.[34]

Thus, Henry the transcendentalist!

Finally with regard to the development of Henry's own aesthetic and his relationship to Laforgue mention should be made of the latter's essay on Impressionism,[35] written in 1883

---

published some four years later, writes to Henry: "Understand that I have devoured your Lespinasse. It is very full and very complete without a doubt. You are indeed a devotee of hers, but look out for your dignity." Laforgue, too, was amazed at Henry's devotion and bizarre attraction to Mlle Lespinasse and at the love ideal with which Henry imbued his fantasy.

34. From the "Étude sur Mademoiselle de Lespinasse," p. 34, in the *Lettres inédites*. Henry dates the study August, 1882. Although some of the writers in the "Hommage à Henry" refer to the fact that Henry loved life, including women, Henry's devotion to Mlle Lespinasse and by extension, Sappho and St. Theresa, is the only real evidence of any love affair on Henry's part. If this is so, one must conclude that Henry was a thoroughly transcendental figure!

35. This essay, originally begun as a statement on works by Pissarro, Degas, and Renoir at the Gurlitt gallery in Berlin in October, 1883, was first published in the *Mélanges posthumes, Oeuvres complètes* (Paris, 1903–4) 3:133–45. William Jay Smith published the English translation in *Art News* 55 (May, 1956):43–45, also in Smith, *Writings of Laforgue*, pp. 190–97, and republished in Linda Nochlin, *Impressionism and Post-Impressionism, 1874–1904* (New York, 1966), pp. 14–20. As Miss Nochlin notes, Laforgue's double interest in art and science must have found an enthusiastic echo in his friendship with Charles Henry, "that remarkably versatile student of science and art . . . who, like the young Laforgue, attempted a kind of synthesis of all fields of human sensibility, thought and action, science and art." My quotes from Laforgue's essay will be from Miss Nochlin's text.

when Laforgue was in Germany, while corresponding with Henry on a large scale. Laforgue had a marked historical interest in art and attended the lectures of Taine at the École des beaux arts in 1880; however, Taine's fixed sociological approach was not to Laforgue's taste or passion. At this same time, while cultivating his friendship with Henry, Laforgue also began to work for Charles Ephrussi of the *Gazette des beaux arts;* Ephrussi himself was something of a promoter of the impressionist painters, certainly one of the first to signal an "official" interest in the new art movement. Be that as it may, in light of the tone that Laforgue adopts in his essay on impressionism, credit must certainly be granted to the very strong possibility of Henry's influence on the ideas put forth in Laforgue's account of impressionism. This must be said particularly in view of Henry's "scientific aesthetic" of 1885 which in many ways is a mathematical refinement of what is expressed in Laforgue's essay written two years prior, though published posthumously in 1903. We may also infer from the many references in Laforgue's letters that Henry was well acquainted with both the art of the salon and the art of the impressionists, not to mention the art of the past.

In any case the chief merit of Laforgue's statement on the new painters is that it is the first recognition of what may be called the psychophysical nature of the impressionist experiment. In his task of defining the impressionist idea, Laforgue draws freely upon the ideas of Helmholtz, Hartmann, and Darwin.[36] By indicating the basically scientific nature of the

36. As early as December, 1882, Laforgue comments to Henry that, "I'm doing, in order to be translated in a review, an article explaining Impressionism to these people [the Germans] who will then say that Impressionism—with all its madness—was born in Germany of Fechner's law" (*Oeuvres*, 4:212). There is an acute truth to this, though there is no reason to believe that Monet was ever acquainted with Fechner's ideas. Also in letter 80 to Charles Ephrussi, dated December, 1883, Laforgue writes, "Have I told you that in these twenty days, locked in and cloistered in this castle of Coblentz, I have thought and worked infinitely? I have re-read the diverse aesthetics of Hegel, Schelling, Saisset, Leveque, Taine—in a mental state that I have not known since I was eighteen years old at the biblio. na-

The Guardian Angel

impressionist vision, Laforgue emphasizes the break with traditional art, which is the victim of its own creation, the academic studio. Laforgue understands that *there can be no
truly visual art that does not take into account the properties
and function of vision:* this can be taken as a fundamental
assumption of the psychophysical aesthetic. Thus Laforgue
states the three "supreme illusions"[37] of traditional painting:
line, perspective, studio lighting, all of which reduce art and
experience to an artificial exercise having little to do with the
actual phenomena of vision. To this, naturally enough, Laforgue offers the alternative of the "impressionist eye," the
product of evolutionary development or, rather, the latest
refinement in the process of seeing:

> Essentially the eye should know only luminous vibra-
> tion, just as the acoustic nerve knows only sonorous
> vibration. The eye, after having begun by appropriat-
> ing, refining, and systematizing the tactile faculties, has
> lived, developed, and maintained itself in this state of
> illusion by centuries of line drawings; and hence its
> evolution as the organ of luminous vibration has been
> retarded in relation to that of the ear, and in respect to
> color harmonics like an auditory prism, the eye sees
> light only roughly and synthetically and has only vague
> powers of decomposing it in the presence of nature,
> despite the three fibrils described by Young,[38] which

---

tionale. I gathered myself, and in one night, from 10 til 4 in the morning,
like Jesus in the Garden of Olives, Saint John on the Isle of Patmos, Plato
on Cape Sunium, Buddha under the fig tree of Gaza [sic], I have written
in ten pages the principle metaphysics of the new Aesthetic, an aesthetic
which accords with the Unconscious of Hartmann, the Transformism of
Darwin, the works of Helmholtz" (ibid., 5:60). This is absolutely fascinating, particularly the interpretation of Darwin's ideas not as evolution, but
as "transformism."
    37. Laforgue, "Impressionism," in Nochlin, *Impressionism,* p. 15.
    38. I draw the reader's attention to the article written by Charles
Henry, "L'Oeuvre ophthalmologique de Thomas Young," *Revue Blanche*
8:473–77. Young (1773–1829), another all-around genius, whom Henry
compares to Newton, was the first in recent times to suggest that the

71

constitute the facets of the prism. The natural eye—or a refined eye, for this organ, before moving ahead, must first become primitive again by ridding itself of tactile illusions—a natural eye forgets tactile illusions and their convenient dead language of line, and acts only in its faculty of prismatic sensibility. It reaches a point where it can see reality in the living atmosphere of forms, decomposed, refracted, reflected by beings and things, in incessant variation. Such is the first characteristic of the Impressionist eye.[39]

This is a statement of incredible depth and insight, combining as it does an essential understanding of evolution, optics, and art history in order to account not only for the development of the impressionist technique as it already existed by the time Laforgue had written his essay, but also taking into account the steps necessary for the further development of art by predicating the necessity of the eye's becoming primitive again. Obviously, for the eye to become "primitive" again, the mind must also become "primitive," but here the concept of primitive can be understood in the sense of shedding the prejudices of acquired knowledge in order to develop further the organs that need development. In this way we can begin to glimpse the evolutionary value of the impressionist movement in the last half of the nineteenth century not only for artistic innovation, but for artistic codevelopment of visual and, by extension, psychic necessity, that

---

three basic color components—"Young's fibrils"—reside not in outside nature, but in the constitution of man's neurophysiological makeup. Though this idea has been modified, it is still an essential truth in modern optics. See Ronchi, L'Optique; R. L. Gregory, Eye and Brain (New York, 1966), pp. 117ff; and Birren, Color Psychology pp. 220–21. Though today this idea is commonly known as the Young-Helmholtz theory, Henry states that there is a definite difference between Young and Helmholtz, in that the former is a "nativist," believing in the existence of fundamental, irreducible instincts, whereas Helmholtz tends towards an "empiricist" point of view, that is, the ultimate explicability of all phenomena.

39. Nochlin, Impressionism, p. 16.

is, the necessity of seeing purely. Laforgue has a profound grasp of the extent to which art shapes and prejudices our vision; certainly the bewilderment with which impressionist painting was received in the nineteenth century is a case in point. Since the eye had been educated to see in terms of line, perspective, and studio lighting, as Laforgue rightly points out, the impressionist painting could only appear as it did to the outraged public and defenders of art. With impressionism, art enters the domain of experimental science, and this, according to the dualistic culture of nineteenth-century Western civilization, was anathema, a veritable confounding of the basic Cartesian categories of science as the observation of "objective" external phenomena (*matter* as it came to be called) and art, the principal expression of the "objectively" unobservable and thus emotionally charged area of mind. Impressionism was a psychovisual bombshell.

In setting off the "academic eye" from the "Impressionist eye," as Laforgue refers to the two fundamentally different modes of visual perception, the poet proclaims that "the Impressionist eye is, in short, the most advanced eye in human evolution, the one which until now has grasped and rendered the most complicated combinations of nuances known."[40] This is because the impressionist "sees and renders nature as it is, that is wholly in the vibration of color. No line, light, relief, perspective, nor chiaroscuro, none of these childish classifications: all these are in reality converted into the vibration of color, and must be obtained on canvas solely by the vibration of color."[41] Laforgue perhaps attributed more to the impressionist idea than even the painters themselves were aware of, but then, Laforgue is writing in 1883, well after the initial impact of the painters had first been felt, and what is expressed in his statements, with their strong emphasis on the scientific understanding of the visual process, should also be regarded as an anticipation of the neo-impressionist paint-

40. Ibid., p. 17.
41. Ibid.

73

ers. Certainly, when Laforgue speaks of the "development of the painter's optic sensibility," he is speaking a language that would be well understood by Seurat or Fénéon, even more so by Charles Henry. And in his description of a painter before a landscape Laforgue displays an amazing optic sensibility:

> In the course of these fifteen minutes [before the landscape], the optical sensibility of the painter has changed time and time again, has been upset in its appreciation of the constancy and relative values of the landscape tones. Imponderable fusions of tone, opposing perceptions, imperceptible distractions, subordinations and dominations, variations in the force of reaction of the three optical fibrils one upon the other and on the external world, infinite and infinitisimal struggles.
>
> One of a myriad examples: I see a certain shade of violet; I lower my eyes toward my palette to mix it and my eye is involuntarily drawn by the white of my shirt sleeve; my eye has changed, my violet suffers. . . .
>
> So in short, even if one remains only fifteen minutes before a landscape, one's work will never be the real equivalent of the fugitive reality, but rather the record of the response of a certain unique sensibility to a moment which can never be reproduced exactly for the individual, under the excitement of a landscape at a certain moment of its luminous life which can never be identified.[42]

What a precise statement of the problem confronting a painter like Seurat at the exact moment in time prior to that painter's preparation for the painting of the *Grande Jatte!* It is not surprising that the intermediary between the sensibility of Laforgue and that of Seurat should have been Charles Henry, who more or less formulated the "solution" or basis upon which an art could be founded not subject to a "fugitive reality" of fleeting impressions. It is here that Henry and

42. Ibid., pp. 17–18.

The Guardian Angel

Seurat part company with Laforgue, who, at the bidding of the great unconscious, would choose to let matters be, in a final paroxysm of individualism, from an excess of which the impressionist painters themselves suffered. But then it was inherent in their approach and technique, a fact of which Laforgue was, once again, so well aware. Thus he states:

Each man is, according to his moment in time, his racial milieu and social situation, his moment of individual evolution, a kind of keyboard on which the exterior world plays in a certain way. My own keyboard is perpetually chanting and there is no other like it. All keyboards are legitimate. The exterior world likewise is a perpetually changing symphony (as is illustrated by Fechner's law, which says that the perception of differences declines in inverse proportion to their intensities). The optical arts spring from the eye and solely from the eye. There do not exist anywhere in the world two eyes identical as organs or faculties.[43]

And in anticipation of the heady atmosphere that was to surround the rise of neo-impressionism and symbolism, Laforgue writes:

The atmosphere favorable to the freedom of this evolution lies in the suppression of schools, juries, medals . . . and in the encouragement of a nihilistic dilettantism and open-minded anarchy like that which reigns amid French artists today: Laissez faire, laissez passer. Law beyond human concerns must follow its automatic pattern, and the wind of the Unconscious must be free to blow where it will.[44]

It is the virtue of Laforgue's thesis concerning impressionism that it shows how the movement, in addition to containing the seeds of its own destruction—the ultimate helplessness of remaining a victim of the moment, the lot of unguided

43. Ibid.
44. Ibid., p. 19.

Chapter Four

labor exemplified in this instance by the brilliant but undirected course of the impressionist painters—also contains the seeds for that which can grow beyond the anarchistic spasms of the unconscious. In his clarity in describing the impressionist situation, Laforgue literally clears the field, and the truth of what he states is easily an assumption or groundwork from which others can build, though not necessarily in the direction foreseen by Laforgue. Almost as if by cue, Henry constructs his edifice in the direction of consciousness, though not without utilizing the fundamental idea set forth by Laforgue, except that Henry explicitly expands the psychophysical assumption contained in Laforgue's essay: *there can be no art, that does not take into account the properties and functions of the various sense organs to which the particular art appeals.*

In summing up, the relation between Henry and Laforgue was clearly of the greatest importance for the development of both young men, in many ways so distinctly opposite in temperament. Yet in these two, because of a great similarity of interests, opposition was turned into a complementarity. Henry was obviously of the greatest encouragement to Laforgue while the latter was in Germany, and, along with Gustave Kahn, Henry attended and aided the publication of Laforgue's first book of verse, *Les Complaintes.* This in itself would gain any poet's lifelong esteem.

But how is one to assess Henry's side of the relationship? By the time the two met, probably in 1879, Henry, though only twenty years old, had distinguished himself with the publication of some half-dozen erudite articles concerning the history of science and mathematics. Henry's nature was markedly philosophical and precise. His friendship with Laforgue most certainly broadened Henry's interests (though at this point it is not clear how much of his artistic or aesthetic interests were due to Laforgue); for while Henry seems to have had some curiosity in this direction when he first came into contact with Laforgue, as in the instance of Henry's in-

The Guardian Angel

troducing Laforgue to the salon of the strange Sandah Mahali, Laforgue at the time was studying art history. Henry's first "art historical" publication dates from 1880—the publication of the documents by Charles Nicholas Cochin concerning the eighteenth-century artists. Is it because of Laforgue that Henry begins to publish art historical material? We do not know for sure, but certainly the intimacy which Henry shared with Laforgue at this time—1879–81—an intimacy seemingly rare for Henry, must have had some bearing on this broadening of Henry's erudite field of interests. Since Laforgue even reminisces in some of the letters to Henry about the times spent in the library, one could even surmise that it was in precisely such situations that Henry's interest turned more specifically to the problem of art.

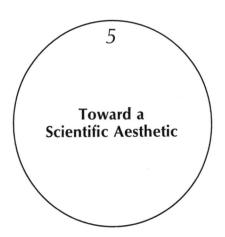

5

Toward a
Scientific Aesthetic

HENRY'S uniqueness, erudite exuberance, and youth guaranteed him a certain popularity, and by the mid-1880s he was giving his well-attended lectures on aesthetics.[1] Certainly these lectures, during which Henry filled a little blackboard with equations and figures and in which he used dress-mannequins draped with varicolored cloths in order to illustrate points in the theory of colors, were developed as part of a program, the articulation of a scientific aesthetic. These lectures were attended by Seurat, Signac, Pissarro, and others.[2] At the same time, Henry continued his scholarly publications. In January of 1885, in fact, about a half-year prior to the publication of the *Esthétique scientifique,* Henry published the manuscripts A and B of Leonardo da Vinci. These manuscripts are not without significance for the development of the art of Seurat and Signac, for in them there is

1. Apparently Henry was eager to lecture on his new theories. As early as 1884 he was lecturing at the Sorbonne; later in the offices of *La vogue* and *L'indépendant.* See Lövgren, *Modernism,* p. 40, and Gustave Kahn, "Charles Henry in "Hommage à Henry," p. 60.

2. The best description of Henry's "school" is given by Georges Lecomte, *Camille Pissarro* (Paris, 1922), p. 75, who describes how the lectures went over Pissarro's head but how Seurat patiently drank them in and later explained them to Pissarro. On the other hand, it is not clear how or when Henry met Signac and Seurat.

A Scientific Aesthetic

much discussion of the problem of reflections and contrasts, an idea of the greatest importance for neo-impressionism, as well as one which becomes central to Henry's entire system.[3]

Though the knowledge of the science of the contrast of colors had "progressed" since Leonardo made his observations, it was one of the problems which Seurat had to cope with in the *Grande Jatte*. It does not seem probable that Henry would have missed the coincidence when he made the artist's acquaintance late in 1885 or early 1886. Another possible connection between Henry and the art scene of the 1885–86 period is the appearance of the so-called "papier de Gauguin," a curious text of the Persian poet Vehbi Mohammed Zunbul-Zade. The reason I conjecture that there is a connection between this document and Henry is because it is from Kahn that we have news of it: "Seurat was concerned about the so-called papier de Gauguin. He [Seurat] possessed a copy of it, for Gauguin did not hide the truth; it was an extract of an oriental text on the coloring of carpets and contained facts on the gradation of harmonies."[4] As I have noted,

3. Consider the following observation by Leonardo: "If you are representing a white body let it be surrounded by ample space, because as white has no color of its own it is tinged and altered in some degree by the color of the objects surrounding it. If you see a woman dressed in white in the midst of a landscape, that side which is towards the sun is bright in color, so much so that in some portions it will dazzle the eyes like the sun itself; and that side which is towards the atmosphere, luminous through being interwoven by the sun's rays and penetrated by them since the atmosphere itself is blue, that side of the woman's figure will appear steeped in blue. If the surface of the ground about her be meadows and if she be standing between a field lighted up by the sun itself, you will see every portion of those folds which are towards the meadows tinged by the reflected rays with the color of that meadow. Thus the white is transmuted into the colors of the luminous and nonluminous objects near it" (*Notebooks*, ed. Irma A. Richter [London, 1959], pp. 138–39). Obviously Henry would be able to amplify such an observation according to the most modern optical theories of Helmholtz, Rood, and Sutter.

4. Gustave Kahn, "Pointillisme," p. 16. Ferté is also mentioned by Laforgue in a letter to Henry dated January 4, 1882. See also Paul Gauguin, *Intimate Journals* (London, 1923), pp. 31–33, and Homer, *Seurat*, pp. 130–31, who considers the Zunbul-Zade text as instrumental in the creation of the *Grande Jatte*.

Chapter Five

Henry, according to Kahn, was in close contact with a certain gentleman, perhaps M. Ferté, who was a translator of Persian verse; on the other hand, there is no evidence that Henry was ever in contact with Gauguin.

Yet it is a curious coincidence that as early as January, 1885, in a letter to Emile Schnuffenecker, one of the founders, along with Signac, of the Salon des Indépendants, Gauguin employs a language and concepts that are most reminiscent of Henry, particularly when we keep in mind that this was the time of Henry's popular lectures on aesthetics. Gauguin writes:

> All our five senses reach the brain *directly,* affected by a multiplicity of things, and which no education can destroy. Whence I conclude there are lines that are noble and lines that are false. The straight line reaches to infinity, the curve limits creation, without reckoning the fatality of numbers. Have the figures 3 and 7 been sufficiently discussed? Colors, although less numerous than lines, are still more explicative by virtue of their potent influence on the eye. There are noble sounds, others that are vulgar; peaceful and consoling harmonies, others that provoke by their audacity. You will find in graphology the traits of candid men and those of liars; why should not lines and colors reveal also the more or less grand character of the artist. . . . The young Raphael knew all these things intuitively and in his pictures there are harmonies of line which cannot be accounted for; they are the veiled reflections of the innermost recesses of the man's mind. . . . The equilateral triangle is the most firmly based and the perfect triangle. A long triangle is more elegant. We say lines to the right advance, those to the left retreat. . . .[5]

The similarity between Gauguin's ideas here and Henry's at this time is phenomenal; as Lövgren notes, Gauguin's letter

5. The letter is dated 14 January, 1885, quoted in Nochlin, *Impressionism*, pp. 158–59.

A Scientific Aesthetic

is like an echo of Henry's lectures on experimental psychology.[6] Indeed, it was Kahn's claim that the symbolical transcendental theory of art could be verified and confirmed by Charles Henry's scientific aesthetic, which was conceived as an instrument that would enable an artist "to break through the veil of empiricism into a crystal-clear world of absolute beauty."[7]

The publication of Henry's *Introduction à une esthétique scientifique* in August, 1885,[8] marks a most significant turning point in the artistic climate of Paris in the last quarter of the nineteenth century. A statement of principles and concepts of great clarity and of a far-reaching nature, the *Esthétique* signals the conscious beginning of the symbolist era. In 1886, along with Gustave Kahn and Félix Fénéon, Henry cofounded the short-lived but influential symbolist journal *La vogue*. Henry became the friend of poets, artists, and presumably musicians as well—Seurat, Signac, Valéry, Mallarmé, to name the most important—whose work benefited from or corresponded to Henry's mathematically organized symbolism.

Scientific dilettante, symbolist brain-trust, aesthetic fountainhead, Henry, in his thought and work during this period, embraces and directs all artistic activity within a program whose sense of harmony and unity go beyond to a social vision whose utopianism is as positivist as it is metaphysical,

6. Lövgren, *Modernism*, p. 93.
7. Ibid., p. 69. Kahn, in the famous "Réponse des symbolistes," states that "Symbolism is the adherence of literature to scientific theories constructed by induction and controlled by the experimentation of M. Charles Henry, announced in an introduction to mathematical and experimental aesthetic philosophical principle which makes us reject all reality of matter and admit the existence of the world only as representation." We have already spoken of how Henry refers to "matter" or the material aspect of things as "representation" in the *Cercle chromatique*. The obvious source for this idea is Schopenhauer who was, of course, the first modern European thinker to express the influence of Buddhist thought.
8. First published in *Revue contemporaine* (August 25, 1885), pp. 441–69.

and which certainly responds to the socialist-anarchist tendencies of the leading artists and thinkers of the period. Indeed, it is my contention that Henry's influence in this period is of the greatest value and importance, more so than that of any other single nonartistic personality active *au temps du symbolisme.*[9] Certainly this holds true for the way in which he helped shape the neo-impressionist painters. Fénéon, the neo-impressionists' "critic," himself derived his major scientific ideas from Henry, and this must be remembered when reading Fénéon's statements on neo-impressionism.[10] In fact neo-impressionism can be seen as a collaboration between scientific theorists (Henry), critic-litterateurs (Fénéon), and painters (Seurat, Signac). But of this, more later.[11]

In the *Esthétique,* Henry at the outset articulates the epistemological situation. According to him there are two ways of understanding:

1. Natural philosophy—what is commonly understood as science (objective understanding).
2. Art (subjective understanding).

In formulating this twofold approach to understanding, Henry obviously draws upon his thorough knowledge of Descartes and the Cartesian system with its dualistic effect upon

9. Indeed, the only other writer in recent times to take this position is Sven Lövgren, who acknowledges the importance of psychophysical research in France with regard to the symbolist movement and who gives to Henry a key role in the formation of modernism (*Modernism,* pp. 41, 66–75).

10. Fénéon first mentions the importance of the work of Henry with regard to the neo-impressionists in the article significantly entitled "L'Impressionnisme scientifique," in *L'Art moderne* (September 19, 1886), in which Fénéon mentions the theory of contrast, rhythm and measure. In *La Cravache* (May 18, 1889), (in Fénéon *Oeuvres,* Paris, 1948, pp. 167–172), Fénéon devotes an entire article, "Une esthétique scientifique," to the work of Charles Henry, with particular reference to the *Cercle chromatique* and the *Rapporteur esthétique,* in which Fénéon relates some of Henry's experiments with colored glasses in determining the directions of colors.

11. In fact this triumvirate of theorist, critic, and artist is apotheosized in the *Portrait of Félix Fénéon,* which I shall discuss in chapter 7.

A Scientific Aesthetic

the culture and mentality of modern Europe, though obviously Henry does not see these two areas as unalterably distinct or separate. The point of his aesthetic is precisely to bridge the supposed gap.

Then Henry formulates what constitutes art and what constitutes aesthetics:

> We will say that art pursues the expression of the *physiognomy of things,* and that aesthetics studies the conditions in which these things are satisfying; that is, when they are represented gay or sad, agreeable or disagreeable, beautiful or ugly. There is not yet an aesthetic of tastes or smells, nor arts which correspond to them. Aesthetic things for us are reduced to forms, to colors, and to sounds.[12]

The tendency on Henry's part to view reality in terms of opposites is most pronounced and is eventually formulated into his principle of dynamogeny and inhibition; it should not be taken as a dualistic attitude such as that implicit in Descartes' concept of mind and matter. On the contrary, there is in Henry's thought a profoundly unitive effort to go beyond mere dualism. For Henry the formulation of opposites is not a conflictive view but one of complementarity. Just as Fechner saw mind and matter as simply two ways of viewing the same phenomena—inner-outer, dayview-nightview—so for Henry the two principles are *complementary* aspects whose total functioning create a unity, much in the manner of the

12. "Une esthétique scientifique," p. 441. With regard to the art of smells and tastes, Fénéon writes in the article "Une esthétique scientifique," "We await the symbolism of tastes and smells. The demonstration [in Henry's method] until now refused by science, of a connection of harmonies among all the senses, we now finally have." This typically symbolist fascination is pursued by Henry in an article entitled "A travers les sciences et les arts," *Revue blanche* (one of whose editors, incidentally, was Félix Fénéon) 6 (1894):254–58, in which Henry discusses artificial perfumes as stimulants whose effects can be determined in much the same manner as the effects of forms or sounds in terms of dynamogeny and inhibition; indeed it is this kind of investigation that led Henry into experimentation with various stimulants and drugs, chief among them kola.

Taoist yin and yang, heaven and earth. Furthermore, a similar way of wording is to be found in Seurat's famous letter to Maurice de Beaubourg of 1890, indicating the extent to which the painter was imbued with Henry's principles.

Then, almost as if in response to Laforgue's own scientific aesthetic which leaves the artist as an isolated individual to the whims and *impressions* of the passing moment, Henry makes the following statement:

> That which science can and must do is to expand the agreeable within us and outside of us, and from this point of view its social function is immense in this time of oppression and blind conflicts. It ought to spare the artist hesitations and useless attempts in assigning or indicating the way in which he can find ever more rich aesthetic elements; it ought to furnish the critic a rapid means of discerning the ugly, so often informulable, however much it is felt.[13]

Here Henry formulates a distinct function for art, a function which, naturally enough, ought to determine the nature and appearance of the given work of art. Like science, art must "expand the agreeable within us and outside of us." Therefore, the work of art must present a harmony, and harmony is, finally, a very precise matter—precise in its constituent elements and in what it purveys. Implicit in this view is something of an evolutionary concept, that of expansion in a definite direction towards the goal of harmony, which can only be achieved through the application of harmony in order to create, within and without, a more agreeable state or condition. It is important once again, to note Henry's assumption that the effect must be felt and witnessed both outside and within. This is the basic psychophysical assumption: no physical action without attendant psychic reaction, and vice versa. Also in Henry's evolutionary assumption there is present what can be called a teleological element that is not necessarily an

13. "Les sciences et les arts," p. 442.

A Scientific Aesthetic

aspect of Darwin's concept of evolution. Finally, there is the emphatic eschewing of the *ugly,* an element for which there is no room in the construction of harmony.[14]

Henry's views are a strange blend of mathematical idealism and rigorous scientific application. Henry is indeed a modern Pythagoras; the world for him is number, and number the revelation of a mystic order. This is why harmony is so important for Henry, as well as for Seurat, because harmony is number visibly manifest; thus, the contemplation of harmony—the properly executed work of art—has a revelatory function. This may account for the reason why what we call spiritual art is so often of such a symmetrical and even geometric nature, for only in this way can the viewer grasp the sense of total order which underlies the religious experience which carries with it intimation of a much more immense order or system of things than is encompassed by mere objective reason. Indeed, Henry is well based in the history of harmony. This history, however, according to Henry, remains on a basically speculative level of operation from the ancient Greeks—Pythagoras, Plato, Aristotle—through Leonardo, Michelangelo, Lomazzo, Rameau, and Hogarth. Here it should be made clear that Henry's concept of "science" is ambiguous. On the one hand he is aware of the shortcomings of the dualistic philosophy of matter which is part and parcel of the normal or classical scientific process, and he endeavors to overcome this attitude, *but by the most rigorously mathematical of means.* In this respect, Henry is very much like Fechner. On the other hand, Henry has a tendency to value according to the very system which he ultimately wishes to transcend; yet it is not clear whether Henry is actually indicating that there was no good theory or study of harmony until the advent of a scientific system in the nine-

14. It is well to recall Laforgue's interpretation of Darwin's idea as "transformism" (see above, chapter 4, n. 36), which is certainly the idea Henry mathematically expresses towards the close of the *Cercle chromatique* as an "indefinitely evolutive principle."

Chapter Five

teenth century, or whether he merely means to say that the only adequate concept of harmony for the particular period is a scientific one, not that such a one is any better than previous ones. At best Henry's position is probably one of evolutionary necessity which recognizes a hierarchical order of development. Thus the only science of harmony that answers the needs of a technological situation is one which takes into account the development of what in the West has come to be called science, with the understanding, of course, that such a system of harmony would be applicable only so long as the system of science which is practiced continues its dominion.[15]

15. Henry's method of transcending the limitations of the dominant system by utilizing the very vocabulary of that system is most reminiscent of the Sufic method described by Ibn-Al-Arabi: "The Sufi must act and speak in a manner which takes into consideration the understanding, limitations and dominant concealed prejudices of his audience," quoted in Idreis Shah, *Special Problems in the Study of Sufi Ideas* (London, 1966), p. 28. A further special study in Sufi ideas might be the consideration: was Charles Henry a Sufi? Idreis Shah, certainly the world's leading expert on the history and philosophy of this historically persistent sect (see also by the same writer, *The Sufis,* Introduction by Robert Graves [New York, 1964]), states that, broadly speaking, "We may call Sufi ideas 'a psychology' " (*Sufi Ideas,* p. 8). Though the Sufis are often associated with Persian poets like Omar Khayyam or Jalaludin Rumi, Shah has proven, without a doubt, a tremendous influence of Sufism in the West, and, in fact, many of the alchemists, religious thinkers of a more heretical nature, and even scientists reflect the impact of Sufic ideas. I have several times referred to a certain M. Ferté, translator of Persian texts and master of languages with whom Henry was in contact in the late 1870s and early 80s—certainly he could have introduced Henry to the basic ideas of Sufism, which can be described as a kind of "transformism," to use Laforgue's mystical interpretation of Darwin. Thus the thirteenth-century Persian poet Rumi writes: "Man is a product of evolution. He continues this process. But the 'new' faculties for which he yearns (generally unknowingly) come into being only as a result of necessity. In other words, he now has to take a part in the development of his own evolution. 'Organs come into being as a response to necessity. Therefore increase your necessity' " (idem, p. 50). A more "transformist" idea would be difficult to find. It would be worthwhile, though probably not very fruitful, to attempt to prove the supposition that Henry was indeed a Sufi, since anonymity is a chief characteristic of Sufis; for, to quote Rumi once again, "those who have developed the 'higher perceptions' sometimes have to conceal this fact, for social and

A Scientific Aesthetic

In any case, for Henry a truly scientific system of harmony is inaugurated in 1827 with the publication in Leyden of the *Essai sur les signes inconditionels dans l'art,* by the Belgian Humbert de Superville. As Henry notes, de Superville's three schematic faces had already been popularized by Charles Blanc,[16] and, as Homer points out, these faces show up in the work of Seurat. Curiously enough, Henry believes that, in addition to the fact that de Superville applied his schema to architecture, a similar system was used and applied by Edgar Allan Poe to literature. Where Henry got this idea is not clear; perhaps from Baudelaire. Certainly Henry's knowledge of Poe must have been through the medium of Baudelaire's translations of Poe and his essay on Poe. Henry's attitude toward Baudelaire is much in the tradition of the symbolists, as might be expected, and later, in the *Esthétique scientifique,* Henry comments on Baudelaire. Following de Superville's *Essai,* Henry cites the work of a certain Comte Durutte, *Esthétique musicale,* published in 1855.[17] Henry also cites the

---

other reasons, behind a socially acceptable facade." Even so, it is well to recall Henry's fate at the hands of the "savants officiels" in the very last years of his life, when Henry's research had poked through the "socially acceptable facade" of *proper* reason. And as a last hint, in the *Théorie du Rayonnement,* p. 100, while discussing the simultaneous excitation of genital and electromagnetic sensations which provoke the equivalent of a psychophysiological "white" defined in literary language as "love," Henry refers these intense internal sensations of nervous exaltation to the well-known practices of the Dervishes, certainly one of the most famous of Sufic cults.

16. "Une esthétique scientifique," pp. 443–44. On the other hand Henry attributes to Rameau the credit of having pushed to its furthest limits, prior to the nineteenth century, the idea or *expression* of a scientific aesthetic. The text by Blanc to which Henry refers is, of course, the *Grammaire des arts du dessin* (Paris, 1867).

17. "Une esthétique scientifique," p. 444. Durette was a disciple of the Polish scientist and mathematician Wronski, who was apparently a great influence on Henry, but about whom there is little information. According to Gustave Kahn, "Hommage à Henry," p. 58, Henry was quite taken—"passionné"—by the figure of Wronski. Indeed, Kahn relates what can be taken as a psychological insight into Henry's character. "Was there not some echo of childhood, of the remembrance of dear Balzac, read and

work of Zeising, Fechner, Wundt, and Hermann from Germany, as well as the work in England of Hay. More significantly, Henry comments on the work of various other researchers—Lagout, Rochas, and, above all, Hanslick and Geroult, the last two of whom addressed themselves to the problem of movement in the aesthetic sensation.[18] Henry's scholarly survey of the development of a scientific aesthetic concludes with consideration of the more psychological approach of Charles Leveque, Sully-Prudhomme, and the works of Mathis Lussy on "expression." In addition, Henry sees an analogous development, towards the more scientific understanding, taking place among the critics and culminating in Taine. And finally Henry states, "I scarcely have need to recall how much the art of Edgar Allan Poe and Charles Baudelaire has exalted science."[19]

Having concluded his historical consideration of the concept of a scientific aesthetic, Henry states the situation thus: "The problem of the aesthetic of forms finally comes down to this: which are the lines that are most agreeable?"[20] However, considering that lines are really an abstraction or a synthesis of perceptions of an object, Henry puts forth the notion that *direction* is the reality which lines suppose. This is an important and fundamental idea in Henry's aesthetic, for directions

---

reread by his [Henry's] mother, and probably recounted to him, in the desire of coming to terms with this scholar, a little strange, a little outside of the law, so that he [Henry] declared with warmth and pleasure that Wronski actually appeared anecdotically and somewhat veiled in the work of Balzac?" This is further evident in Henry's book *Wronski et l'esthétique musicale.*

18. What Henry does in effect is give a rundown of the recent psychophysical research, though he is nowhere very explicit with regard to what he derives from each of the scientists that he mentions. The work of Fechner and Wundt is, of course, well known; for the work of Geroult on movement see above, chapter 4, n. 19. Eduard Hanslick, whom Henry later quotes, wrote in 1885 *Vom Musikalisch-Schoenen, Ein Beitrag zur Revision der Aesthetik der Tonkunst* (Leipzig).

19. "Une esthétique scientifique," p. 444.

20. Ibid., p. 445.

A Scientific Aesthetic

are to be understood as psychic phenomena corresponding to the perception of the sensation of a physical nature. Then Henry reformulates his question: "Which are the agreeable directions? Which the disagreeable? Or, said in a different way, which directions do we associate with pleasure and which with pain?"[21] Here again Henry reduces the experience of reality to *two* basic sensations: pleasure and pain, which naturally enough correspond to the two basic psychophysiological motor functions of dynamogeny and inhibition, expansion and contraction, diastole and systole, epitomized in the primary psychophysiological act of breathing—psychophysiological because although breathing is a necessary physiological motor function, the control of breathing is a psychic function.

Citing experiments by Helmholtz, Mantegazza, and Richot, Henry concludes that what distinguishes pleasure from pain is not intensity of sensation, but the continuity or the discontinuity of sensation. Because it takes more effort to maintain the perception of a discontinuous sensation, such sensations create what we call sad or painful reactions; because there is less effort needed to maintain the perception of a continuous sensation, such sensations may be said to create agreeable or pleasurable reactions. After discussing briefly the basic physiological states expressive of pain and pleasure, Henry relates direction to psychophysiological reaction: "In summing up, to pleasure corresponds the direction from low to high; furthermore, it is this which determines the position of the energy which is capable of being utilized by us, the energy which the mechanical theory of heat calls the *energy of position*. To sadness corresponds the direction from high to low; moreover, it is that which determines the position of energy which has lost all its usefulness, *degraded energy*."[22]

Not only does Henry consider the up-down aspect of en-

21. Ibid.
22. Ibid., p. 447.

ergy, but the "horizontal," left-right aspect as well. That direction is agreeable which goes from left to right, and disagreeable which goes from right to left.[23] The effects of these directions, furthermore, are subject to the intensity of the pathological disposition of the subject; to a depressed person, naturally enough, agreeable directions will appear disagreeable. Emphasizing the universality of the principles, Henry states that the theory of correspondence of directions applies equally to color and sound. Finally, with regard to these preliminary observations on directions, Henry indicates that disagreeable directions are *absolutely* all of those lines which are not simple directions, and, relatively, all of those directions contrary to agreeable directions. As a poetic conclusion, Henry cites a certain geometrician, M. Laguerre, who speaks of the "dissonances of line."[24]

What is significant thus far in this brief review of the *Esthétique scientifique* is, on the one hand, its "abstract" nature and therefore its universal applicability to the various arts, which is also another way of indicating the basic unity of the arts, a key synthetist idea echoing the Wagnerian *gesamtkunstwerk;* on the other hand, there is the strong emphasis on the psychic factor of the aesthetic experience. I stress this because it is precisely the "abstract" and psychic nature of the art of the symbolist period, including neo-impressionism, the synthetism of Gauguin, the poetry of Mallarmé, Valéry,

23. Ibid., pp. 447–48. Though Henry is attempting to articulate scientifically the theory of directions with regard to psychophysical reactions in the human organism, he is inevitably drawn into making more cosmic observations. The more agreeable direction, that from left to right, is the direction in which man, at least in the Northern hemisphere, turns to face the sun, and which is the opposite or inverse direction of the turning of the earth; thus the direction left to right simultaneously opposes what can be called the electromagnetic ether and creates a resistance, but it is precisely in this encounter with the electromagnetic ether, this resistance, that consciousness occurs. "Going towards the right, or raising himself," Henry states, "man goes towards the sun and it is without a doubt in the sun, the source of all life, that he must seek the physical reason of the expression which we attribute to the different directions."
24. Ibid., p. 449.

A Scientific Aesthetic

and the curious René Ghil, as well as the music of Debussy, which sets it apart from the previous artistic generation; it should be kept well in mind the extent to which Henry sets forth the basic aesthetic code of the symbolist generation in his *Esthétique scientifique*. Again, it would not be an exaggeration to say that this work sets the tone for what follows. Thus Henry states that although pleasure is the correlative of a minimal perceptual effort, it is expressed by a tendency to realize a maximum amount of work; paraphrasing Descartes, he continues, "the more complex the equation, the more beautiful it is . . . the more complex are the curves, the more beautiful they are."[25] Here we have an intimation of the flowing arabesque and organic lines which are so characteristic of art nouveau, the final visual expression of the symbolist era.

Having established his theory of the correspondence of directions, Henry then moves into a discussion of what may be called the kinesthetic factor, properly summed up in the concept of rhythm. Rephrasing Gauss's principle of least effort, Henry states: "Movement is accomplished during each infinitesimal element of time under the least effort possible."[26] To this Henry appends a further psychophysical consideration: "To the least mechanical effort corresponds, evidently, the least effort of perception."[27] Motion—the kinetic effect—results from a *change of direction,* and "every change of direction is an angle; furthermore every angle is measureable by the arc of a circle, intercepted through its sides, the center of the circle being the summit of the angle."[28] Here for the first time Henry introduces another key idea in his aesthetic: the abstract element of the circle and its kinetic counterpart, the cycle. For Henry, the neo-Pythagorean, the circle and the cycle represent the whole, the complete and irreducible, which contains the fluctuations of the two polar-

25. Ibid., p. 450.
26. Ibid.
27. Ibid.
28. Ibid.

ities of dynamogeny and inhibition, in much the same manner as the Taoist circle-symbol of unity which contains the yin and the yang. Henry continually resorts to the circle as the basic ground whose 360° sum up all possible directions and psychic attitudes. Thus Henry later produces the *Rapporteur esthétique* (based on the circle), *Le Cercle chromatique,* as well as the idea of the cycle of perception which he introduces in his article on "Dynamogeny and Inhibition." As a bicycle enthusiast, Henry's preoccupation with the circle and cycles is carried to its 'pataphysical ultimate in the series of articles on "cyclisme," though even later in his career he uses the circle and circular functions in order to describe his model of the elementary static equilibrium, the *psychone.* In the visual arts the influence of Henry's circular functions is best seen in Seurat's *La Cirque,* and above all, in Signac's *Portrait of Fénéon.*[29] Emphasizing the idealist, Pythagorean strain in his calculations, Henry paraphrases the definition of rhythm as given by Aristides, Quintilian, and Aristoxenes, and as formulated by Charles Leveque: "Rhythm is order in time or measure."[30] Henry then gives the following definition: "We shall thus define rhythm: a change of direction determining on a circumference, of which the center is at the center of change, a possible geometric division, that is to say a division in a number of parts M, which may be 2, 2^n or a number of the form 2^n+1 or the product of a power of 2 by one or several different numbers of this form."[31] Here Henry gives the basic formula which governs the function of the *Cercle chromatique* and the *Rapporteur esthétique,* and lists those numbers which as degrees, correspond to agreeable directions and harmonious divisions of a circle: 2, 3, 4, 5, 6, 8, 10, 12, 15, 16, 17, 20, 24, 30, 32, 34, 40, 48, 51, 60, 64, 80, 85, 96. Defining

29. Robert Delaunay's predilection for the circle, in works around 1912, as well as the *Discs of Newton* by Frank Kupka, of about the same time, may well be related to Henry's ideas. See Dénise Fédit, *L'oeuvre de Kupka* (Paris, 1966), p. 79.
30. "Une esthétique scientifique," p. 451.
31. Ibid., pp. 451–52.

A Scientific Aesthetic

measure as a relation between two terms, Henry is led into a discussion on proportion, culminating, naturally enough, in the formulation of the golden section $(\frac{a}{b} = \frac{b}{a} + b)$. Once again we see how on the one hand Henry is the exponent of a precise, "scientific" aesthetic, but how, on the other hand, this aesthetic is often nothing more than a reformulation of profoundly classical ideas. One should recall here not only Henry's research in the history of mathematics and science, but also his work on the French academics, Cochin, Caylus, Bouchardon, and the brothers Slodtz, as well as the publication of the Leonardo da Vinci manuscripts A and B in January of the same year in which the *Esthétique scientifique* was published. Obviously what Henry stresses in handling the tradition of the classical formulas on proportion is the most abstract element of intellectual harmony. It is this which Henry transmits to Seurat or, better, it is in this highly idealistic conception of proportion that Seurat and Henry find common ground.

Concluding his general discussion on the aesthetic of line (or directions) Henry states, "Each figure being an ensemble of changes of directions, we now possess a theory of agreeable directions, of rhythms and measures; thus, we can evidently trace agreeable figures."[32] In this statement there is a concise key to the formal simplifications and "distortions" of the figures and landscapes of the work of the neo-impressionists dating from the later 1880s and early 1890s, culminating in *La Cirque,* the Fénéon portrait, and the work of Van de Velde.[33] It is well worth noting that essentially all of Henry's

32. Ibid., pp. 453–54.
33. We single out Henri Van de Velde only because he is exemplary as a developer of art nouveau in going from painting to more purely decorative work. It is certainly most significant that, as a painter, Van de Velde was a neo-impressionist during the years when Henry's influence was its strongest on the group, particularly following the publication of the *Rapporteur esthétique* and *Cercle chromatique* towards 1890. It is not difficult to see in Henry's emphasis on line and direction, especially dynamogenous

aesthetic ideas are summed up as early as 1885. What came
in the years following was a further explication both through
lecturing and the written word; indeed, it is in the years from
1885 to 1895 that Henry addresses himself almost exclusively
to the problem of aesthetics. On the other hand it is difficult
to say what exactly were his motivations or, more precisely,
how he conceived the role he was playing.

Having formulated his basic principle of line, direction,
and the component aspects of rhythm and measure, Henry
turns to the problem of color, beginning with an immediate
critique of Chevreul, whose color circle Henry "corrects."
Chevreul's chief failure in Henry's eyes is primarily a mathematical one, that of failing to compute properly the angles
of the color wheel with regard to the areas occupied by the
specific colors. As shall be seen, Henry develops a system of
correspondences which relate directions to colors. Again, according to the fundamental system of complementary polarities, color is divided into two basic emotional ranges: gay—
red, orange, yellow; sad—green, blue, violet. This emotional
assignation obviously applies as well to light and shade.
Henry also views color as a function of space, whereas sound
is a function of time; he cites the studies of Helmholtz and
Rood on this matter, as well as on the subject of the expres-
siveness of color. It need hardly be added here that Seurat
was well aware—perhaps independently of Henry, as Homer
so strongly suggests—of the work of Rood and Helmholtz as
well as that of Chevreul. On the other hand, bringing the

---

directions and lines, a shift from correcting nature in a painting by reducing the forms of nature to certain symbolic and rhythmic directions, to
creating without intermediate reference and in a most direct manner those
dynamogenous lines and directions. An excellent example is Van de
Velde's *Haymaking*, painted around 1893, now in the collection of the
estate of Henri Van de Velde and reproduced in Schmutzler, *Art Nouveau*
(New York, 1964), plate 139. Rewald, *Post-impressionism*, p. 284, mentions that W. Finch executed decorative work according to Henry's
theories.

material together as he does, Henry certainly crystallizes the matter. After commenting on the intrinsically fatiguing qualities of the six basic colors (green, violet, blue, red, orange, yellow, in order of fatigability from most to least), Henry develops his idea of the directions of the colors. Red, for instance, being a very agreeable color, has a direction that goes from low to high, corresponding with the direction which causes pleasure; yellow, the most calming of colors, has a horizontal direction.[34] Accordingly, the concept of the contrast of directions, introduced earlier in his essay, is clarified by the idea of the contrast of colors, already well articulated by Chevreul; and the idea of measure in color is clarified by the concept of the directions of colors. Henry concludes his discussion of color with remarks on the difference between subtractive and additive color mixture; the latter technique, as is well known, was employed extensively by the neo-impressionist painters, and is certainly, along with the technique by which that color was applied, the cause of the white-to-gray overall color quality of many of the neo-impressionist canvases.

What is well to note in this brief discussion of Henry's comments on color in the *Esthétique scientifique* is, again, the extent to which his fundamental ideas are already developed, as well as the way in which the color theory is integrated into the theory of directions. It is the integration of all the various factors involved in the aesthetic experience which is perhaps the most important idea established by Henry, for it is the key to what one may call a "depth har-

34. This is certainly one of the most original ideas developed by Henry, that of different colors corresponding to different psychic directions which can be represented absolutely on a circle—thus the idea of "the chromatic circle." Henry does not use this term in "Une esthétique scientifique," although he does allude to the fact (p. 453) that he will write a future work to be entitled "Principes d'esthétique mathématique et expérimentale." Henry never wrote a work with that title, although the *Cercle chromatique* can certainly be described as such a work.

Chapter Five

mony," a concept which calls into play all the psychophysical faculties, which mutually interact and complement one another in the most harmonious way possible. For this reason it is absolutely necessary to consider the whole of Henry's aesthetic even if one is only interested in its application to the visual arts, for Henry's vision is a peculiarly all-embracing one, with its foundation in the principle of universal integration. Such ideas, forming in many ways the basis of symbolism or synthetism, were quite in harmony with the times, whose vision was epitomized by the *gesamtkunstwerk* of Wagner. One need only look at the program notes to the exhibitions of Les XX in the late 1880s to understand the extent to which the integrative arts idea was put into effect. Perhaps totally aware of or in tune with this idea, Henry saw his role clearly as being an intellectual exemplar promulgating in his own way this fundamental notion of integrative depth harmony. And because the symbolist era was one in which the arts borrowed, or at least emphasized borrowing freely from one another, it is well worth considering the remainder of the *Esthétique scientifique*. For finally, Henry's aesthetic is the aesthetic of synesthesia.[35]

Henry follows his discussion of color with a discussion of sounds, relating immediately the theory of directions to the theory of sounds. He quotes the composer Saint-Saëns, who had recently asked in *La France* (March 23, 1885), why sharp sounds are associated with height and grave sounds with low-

35. For literature on this subject, see H. R. Rookmaaker, *Synthetist Art Theories* (Amsterdam, 1959); more interesting is Marie-Antoinette Chaix, *La correspondance des arts dans la poésie contemporaine* (Paris, 1919), who, though scarcely mentioning Henry, goes into the relation of the psychophysical literature of the period with particular regard to the phenomenon of "audition colorée," often citing the same sources that Henry draws upon, that is, Wundt, *Psychologie physiologique,* published in Paris in 1886, or Feré's study *Sensation et mouvement* (Paris, 1887). Mention should also be made of Elizabeth Puckett Martin, "Symbolist Criticism of Painting in France, 1880–95," Ph.D. dissertation (Bryn Mawr, 1952), who draws together much material touching on the same problem of synesthesia, or the synesthetic effect.

ness.[36] Sound—music—is perhaps even easier to explain by Henry's theory of directions than is form or color. In what is a most apropos comment on the development of the visual arts, as well as music, Henry cites again the works of Hanslick, particularly the analogy that is drawn between music, which offers beautiful forms without having an exact feeling for the subject, and ornamental sculpture. According to Henry, Hanslick formulates a principle of "continual autogenesis," a principle which applies equally to music and ornamental sculpture. This is a most suggestive idea, indicating as it does a rich, organic flow or growth principle which Henry must have found to be totally apposite to his own principle of dynamogenous and inhibitory fluctuations. Furthermore, it is precisely such an idea—continual autogenesis—which, combined with Henry's own integratively organic principles, would seem to form a root concept for the art nouveau which developed in the 1890s.[37] Henry Van de Velde, one of the prime decorative mentalities of the 1890s, began late in the 1880s as a neo-impressionist; it does not seem at all implausible that Van de Velde's germ idea came in part from contact, however indirect, with Henry's ideas, particularly since Van de Velde's employment of the neo-impressionist technique dates from the highpoint of Henry's influence on that group of painters during the time from 1888 to 1891.

Writing further on music, Henry speaks of the attraction of

36. "Une esthétique scientifique," p. 458. This is the same question Henry deals with in his article on the law of the evolution of musical sensation in the *Revue philosophique* in 1886. See above, chapter 3, n. 62.

37. "Une esthétique scientifique," pp. 458–59. Henry gives a lengthy quote from Hanslick which is most suggestive, for the German aesthete speaks of "vibrating lines" which thicken and then turn into gracious curves and so on. "But let us go further," says Hanslick, "and represent the living arabesque as the active radiation of an artistic spirit whose total imagination is passed entirely by incessant labor, through thousands of sensitive fibers: will the experience be not akin to that of music?" Henry agrees wholeheartedly with this description of the continual autogenesis of infinite lines.

sounds as a matter of directions: "Music is the concrete representation of abstract directions, and it is the extreme mobility of each note in the sense of its attraction that harbors the secret of its charm, at once so intellectual and so sensual. . . ."[38] This brings to mind the fact that from early in 1886 to 1892, the painter Signac, who later collaborated with Henry, labelled his paintings with opus numbers; considering the way in which Henry describes the function and quality of the musical note, it is not difficult to see how a painter like Signac would find such statements more than applicable to the handling and function of color and visual form. Further connections between Henry's description of music and the neo-impressionist painters is to be found in Henry's discussion of Helmholtz's theory of musical vibrations. Henry relates that "Helmholtz has demonstrated that timbre depends on the form of the vibrations, and that this form depends on the perceptible presence or absence of certain harmonic tones of the fundamental note. . . ."[39] Again, this description of timbre is altogether analogous to the optical vibration which is the essential technical aspect of neo-impressionism; in a neo-impressionist painting the discussion of timbre could be paraphrased to read as a discussion of the vibratory quality of a certain color-area decomposed into its component factors of tone and value, depending on the local color, its complementary, reflected colors and their complementaries, and so on. This complex factor—light-vibration—could only be translated by the pointillist technique to achieve the proper effect of vibration, resulting in the famous "optical mixture" of the neo-impressionists. Thus, after describing in great detail the technique of the *Grande Jatte*, Fénéon states that the atmosphere is transparent and singularly vibrating.[40] And, of course, Laforgue's description of the Impressionist

38. Ibid., p. 461.
39. Ibid., p. 465.
40. Félix Fénéon, in *Au-dela de l'impressionnisme,* ed. F. Cachin (Paris, 1966), p. 67.

A Scientific Aesthetic

technique utilizes to a great extent the idea of optical vibrations which stems from the works of Helmholtz, whose *Physiological Optics* is such a key work for the visual arts during this period. The point here is that the psychophysiological language employed to describe both auditory and visual phenomena is often the same, and this must be seen as a scientific factor behind the synthesizing of the arts in the 1880s.

"We possess a general theory of rhythm and measure," writes Henry, "it remains for us only to apply it to *all* changes of direction. For by the method of graphs, all phenomena are translatable by changes of direction automatically registered."[41] With the utmost precision Henry formulates the basis, as he so puts it, of translating from one sense organ to another, the simultaneousness of which results in synesthesia and, by extension, facilitates the transition from one art form to another. Henry does this by the technique of translating sense phenomena—vibratory changes—into mathematical equations which can be graphed and scaled so that what is a visual symbol is also auditory, and so on. Essentially, what Henry is formulating is the basis for a universal symbolic system, which he was later to refer to as symbolic calculus. Before concluding his *Esthétique scientifique*, Henry also alludes to the idea that what he is formulating for the visual and auditory arts can also be applied to the literary arts as well, and suggests, following a certain M. Barlow, that there are intrinsic vibratory expressive qualities to vowels and consonants. Thus, there can be a psychophysiologically based poetry, something which Henry feels Baudelaire was aiming at, for instance, in the famous "Correspondances."[42] That Henry should also have extended himself into literary aesthet-

41. "Une esthétique scientifique," p. 466.
42. As Baudelaire wrote in *L'art romantique*, first published in 1885, "The time is not far distant when all literature which refuses to march fraternally between science and philosophy will be a literature of suicide and homicide." Indeed, Henry cites lines from Baudelaire's *Les Fleurs du mal*, as examples of a poetry capable of yielding to his science ("Une scientifique esthétique," p. 467).

Chapter Five

ics should not be too surprising considering his friendship with Laforgue, Kahn, and Fénéon. Nor should it be forgotten that Rimbaud's famous verse, "Vowels," which prefigures Henry's aesthetic ideas, was first published in *La vogue*. The work of René Ghil, whose *Traité du verbe* was first published in 1886–87 and which pursues a "scientific" literary theory and program much like that suggested by Henry, is yet another instance in which Henry's influence is almost certainly a factor.[43] Henry's achievement is that he was able to formulate, with a precision that is astonishing, the entire theory of correspondences, for this is finally what his symbolic calculus comes down to.

"But science will never be able to create beauty," Henry adds, having put forth his theory; "for in order to realize beauty, one must possess the universal formula: but to possess the universal formula, wouldn't that be to know it? And the day when the problem will be close to being solved, will not humanity have returned once again to the unconsciousness of Nature?"[44] Curious and mystical afterthought! so reminiscent of the ideas of Laforgue and Hartmann, containing as it does the germ of an evolutionary concept rich in its implications. Consciousness as it is now experienced is but a middle phase, a transition from one level of "unconsciousness" to another; furthermore, implicit in the concept is the idea that the transitional phase of consciousness, presumably the entire historical period of the race, is the phase in which man is most estranged from nature.[45]

43. However, in 1891 Henry declared that Ghil's approach was unscientific and false. See, "Réponse à l'enquête de Jules Huret sur l'évolution de la littérature française," *L'echo de Paris* (June, 1891).

44. "Une esthétique scientifique," p. 467.

45. Henry is forever the "romantic" scientist, but this must not be taken as a contradictory quality; on the contrary, we can see Henry's type as a necessary link in the creation of a new synthesizing world view which is represented by a merging of certain Eastern as well as Western traditions. As an example of this, and of a conception of the evolutionary function of consciousness similar to that developed by Henry, we draw the reader's attention to Govinda, *Early Buddhist Philosophy*, pp. 89ff., and

A Scientific Aesthetic

What must be emphasized in Henry's aesthetic is this: the vision of the integration of the faculties, the looking forward to a new era of symbolism in which art will express knowledge and knowledge will be the expression of what is universally known and experienced. Certainly Henry was aware of the nature of the problem. It was the purpose of his earlier research to articulate the problem of advanced individual self-consciousness and the consequent fragmentation of the faculties which is accompanied by an increasingly complicated technological and social system. This system is supported by a profoundly dualistic knowledge system—science —and the cultivation of progressively exclusive and aesthetically decadent means of expression—art. Finally emphasizing his evolutionary (rather than merely "scientific") approach, Henry sums up:

> I have said that the agreeable directions from low to high, down to up, and from left to right are found to coincide with the tendencies of man towards the light: why? Place on a table lighted from one side: plasmodium reduced to its essential substance, which is called the protoplasm; the leaves of a sensitive plant; the stamens of a climbing nettle—they all turn towards the light; place these underneath a bell permeated by ether or chloroform, the movements come to a halt.[46] Why? It is this yet mysterious tendency whose function the evolutionary system of the world has to make precise.[47]

On this biological and evolutionary note Henry ends his *Introduction à une esthétique scientifique*, though here, too, his comments, apparently based on experiments by Paul Bert, under whom Henry studied early in his career, bring to mind

---

particularly the diagram on p. 91, "structure and development of consciousness."

46. In the original text, Henry inserts in parentheses at this point the name of Paul Bert, one of the men under whom Henry studied in the late 1870s, an experimental physiologist.

47. "Une esthétique scientifique," pp. 468–69.

Chapter Five

the interest of Laforgue in the work of Hartmann, and also
recall the fact that Fechner, whose ideas in so many ways
Henry seems to follow, wrote a curious piece entitled *Nanna,
Or the Soul Life of Plants* and that Goethe published a treatise on the metamorphosis of plants.[48]

48. Fechner's work was published in 1848 and develops the idea that
from the evident design in their organization, the helpful interaction of
their organs and so forth, it may be assumed that there is a soul in plants
as well as men; obviously this comes near to a pantheistic or mystical
doctrine. Goethe too developed his idea of the *Urpflanze* as a kind of basic
metaphor of the stages of growth which are universally applicable; many
of Goethe's ideas stem from Boehme, who, of course, is one of the classic
Western hermetics. See R. D. Gray, *Goethe the Alchemist* (Cambridge,
1952). Henry never gave up his interest in biology, and it was always a
continuing area of research with him. Thus, in the May 25 issue of the
Revue contemporaine 2 (1885):103–17, just three months prior to the
publication of "Une esthétique scientifique," Henry published an article
entitled "Les microbes de l'atmosphère," which brings the reader up to
date on the then new science of atmospheric micrography. Judging from
the graphs which Henry presents, it is evident that this area of his research
had been going on for some five years prior to this publication.

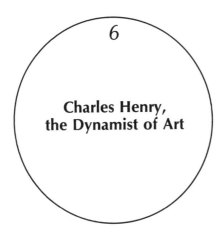

6

Charles Henry,
the Dynamist of Art

AMONG the gentlemen meeting regularly at the Café le
Panier fleuri in the mid-1880s and described by Jules
Christophe as forming the nucleus of the symbolist movement, was Charles Henry, "dynamist of art, future author of
a 'mathematical and experimental aesthetic.' "[1] Also at the
café with Henry were Gustave Kahn ("papadiamantop-
oulos, blue-beard Athenian [pseudonymously called Jean
Moreas]"), Félix Fénéon, Paul Adam, Edouard Dujardin (cre-
ator of the *Revue wagnerienne*), Féodor Fédorowitch de
Wyzewa ("oblomoviste montmartois"), Dubois-Pillet, Seurat,
and Signac ("the painters of an independent touch"), Jules
Laforgue, Maurice Raymond ("statuary polychromist"), and
the curious Barbevara, Italian doctor, pupil of Charcot.[2] As

1. Jules Christophe's description appeared in his article, "Symbolisme,"
La cravache (Paris, June 16, 1888). The description was written just prior
to the publication of the *Cercle chromatique,* and thus the "mathematical
and experimental aesthetic" refers to the title used by Henry in the *Esthétique scientifique* (see above, chapter 5, n. 34).
2. Christophe's curious description is obviously of a situation in 1887
since Laforgue died in August of that year. In addition to the more familiar
symbolist figures, there is the statuary polychromist Maurice Raymond and
the hypnotist Barbevara. Polychrome statuary is a phenomenon Henry concerned himself with as early as 1884, with the publication on ancient techniques of encaustic painting, and is a subject he touches upon in the discussion of color in the *Cercle chromatique;* furthermore, there is Kahn's

Chapter Six

Lövgren observes, the description of the various characters involved in the gatherings at the café are as if taken from the *Deliquescences,* of Adoré Floupette at whose favorite café the symbolists met.[3] Henry is depicted in a situation suggestive of a milieu in which his aesthetic theories found receptivity. If, according to Kahn, the entire "transcendental symbolist aesthetic" can be found in Henry's *Introduction à une esthétique scientifique,* Henry must be understood as a key figure of this group. But how does he effect a correspondence between a "transcendental symbolist aesthetic" and a "mathematical and experimental aesthetic"?

As Kahn suggests, and as has been amply indicated, the *Esthétique scientifique* contains the statement of the aesthetic problem which the symbolist generation faced. In a series of works published shortly after the *Esthétique scientifique,* Henry formulates in some detail the solutions to the aesthetic problem which had in part been posed by himself. Perhaps the most ambitious of these works is the *Cercle chromatique,* in which he spells out at length the basic theories behind his synthesizing aesthetic. Indeed, contained in this work is the essence of ideas that appear in various articles, among them "Contraste, rhythme, et la mesure," "La dynamogénie et l'inhibition," and "L'Esthétique des formes."[4]

---

article, "De l'esthétique du verre polychrome," *La vogue* (April 18, 1886), pp. 54–65.

3. Lövgren, *Modernism,* pp. 63–64.

4. The *Cercle chromatique* was published first as "Cercle chromatique et sensation de couleur," *La revue indépendante* (May, 1888), pp. 238–89. Later that year was published the *Cercle chromatique, présentant tous les compléments et toutes les harmonies de couleurs avec une introduction sur la théorie générale du contraste, du rhythme et de la mesure.* The publisher was Charles Verdin, "constructeur d'instruments de précision pour la physiologie," who also published the *Cercle chromatique* Color Wheel in a large folio, similar in size to that of the *Rapporteur esthétique, permettant l'étude et la rectification de toutes formes avec une introduction sur les applications . . . ,* which was published by G. Seguin, "constructeur d'instruments de précision." The large folio edition of the *Cercle chromatique* was obviously published as a precision instrument and thus contains

The Dynamist of Art

Appearing in separate publications were the *Rapporteur es-thétique* and the *Harmonie des formes et couleurs,*[5] though in many ways these works too are recapitulated and summed up in the *Cercle chromatique* by virtue of its condensed and potent logic. For this reason, in discussing the nature and essence of Henry's aesthetic as it was developed in the symbolist period, the main concern should be in elucidating the contents of the *Cercle chromatique,* with reference where necessary, of course, to other works, and with the intention of presenting Henry's aesthetic as a coherent and organic whole.

In the *Esthétique scientifique,* Henry states:

> The problem of an aesthetic of forms comes down to this: what are the *most agreeable lines?* But a little re-flection shows us quickly that line is an *abstraction:* it is the synthesis of the two parallel and opposite directions in which it is inscribed; the reality is the direction. I do not see a circle: I only see circles inscribed in one direction or in another which one calls "cycles." The problem leads to the conclusion announced: what are the agreeable directions? What are the disagreeable directions? In other words, what directions do we associate with *pleasure* and with *pain?*[6]

Le cercle chromatique begins with a presentation of the theory of directions and its relation to what Henry calls "interior

---

little text. In addition Henry read a paper, "Sur un cercle chromatique, un rapporteur et un triple décimètre esthétiques," *Comptes rendus de l'Aca-démie des Sciences* 18 (January 18, 1889):169–71. Also appearing in the *Comptes rendus de l'Académie des Sciences,* same volume and year, on January 7, pp. 70–71, was a report by Henry "Sur la dynamogenie et L'inhibition."

5. The *Harmonie de formes et de couleurs* (Paris, 1891) was originally given as a number of practical demonstrations of the *Cercle chromatique* and the *rapporteur esthétique* at the Bibliothèque Forney (March 27, 1890).

6. "Une esthétique scientifique," p. 445. Also *Cercle chromatique,* p. 11.

work" or psychic states.[7] This is the psychophysical seed of his aesthetic which simply states that there is a "living mechanics" and that corresponding to the "expression of every mental state and of every idea there is a movement of the body and most especially of the appendages."[8]

Given the fundamental proposition that "every variation of physiological work is represented by changes of directions of energy, be it real or virtual,"[9] Henry sets up the dynamics of his system. Obviously implicit in the idea of direction is a basic dynamics that can be expressed mathematically and kinesthetically. Henry was quite aware of the experimental work of Marey on kinesthetics and rhythm so famously exemplified in his photographs of the figure in motion dating from the period of Henry's own aesthetic experimentation.[10] In a

7. My text is from the extended version of the *Cercle chromatique;* chapter 1 is entitled, "Travail intérieur et directions."

8. "L'esthétique des formes," p. 120. Indeed, Henry's idea of the bio-psychic norm is a circle and its center point, to which are added the various organs or appendages. Thus in the *Cercle chromatique,* Henry states at the outset that "the schematic study of animal mechanics proves that we can describe continuously only complete or partial cycles." The circle and the cycle are the bases of Henry's thought and method.

9. *Cercle chromatique,* p. 14. By "virtual" Henry generally means something like "inner" or idea or thought; there is always some "mental" note made, however unconscious that mental note might be, in response to sensation, or from which results a physiological action; by "real" as opposed to virtual, Henry intends something like "actual." But as it is, the entire psychophysiological apparatus or set-up of such a nature, occurring as it does in time, means that the distinction between causal sensation and psychic effect is not at all distinct.

10. Edouard Marey, 1830–1904, began his photochronographic studies in 1882 in order to determine more exactly the nature of physiological motion. See his *Étude de la locomotion animale par la chronophotographie* (Paris, 1887). Henry makes great use of Marey's research in his own studies of rhythm in the *Cercle chromatique.* It is quite possible also that Marey and Henry were acquainted, if not friends, since their research was of a mutual concern and interest. Both Marey and Henry were to be influential on a later generation of artists who drew from these two psychophysiologists an understanding of the dynamic nature of reality, that is, artists around 1908–14—Cubists, Orphists, Futurists. Aaron Scharf, *Creative Photography* (London, 1965), p. 38, published a chronophotograph by Marey of a subject experimenting with a stationary bicycle apparatus—could this

The Dynamist of Art

transcendental aesthetic, the theory of directions yields two universal direction/reactions: dynamogenous, from left to right and from low to high in a generally clockwise direction; and inhibitory, from right to left and from high to low in a generally counterclockwise direction.[11]

Here then are expressed two of the essentials of Henry's aesthetic:

1. The theory of directions and interior work (psychophysical correspondence)
2. The theory of dynamogeny and inhibition.

It is important to keep these key ideas well in mind in pursuing the rest of Henry's aesthetic, for ulimately all the various psychosensory components have their base in the theory of directions expressed psychophysically as either dynamogenous or inhibitory movement. Furthermore, it can be said that direction is flow, flow is motion, motion is the reality which our senses experience. Undifferentiated flow visually presented is pure light, which is represented as a continuous

headless figure dressed in a white pyjama-like suit be Charles Henry? Scharf dates the photograph ca. 1890; in addition to the mutual physiological rhythm-and-motion research, we must recall Henry's own enthusiasm for bicycling and his own studies on the psychophysiology of this sport in 1894–95. Henry, of course, makes note of Marey's bicycle research, *Revue blanche* 7 (1894):554–61.

11. *Cercle chromatique*, pp. 14ff, "Dynamogenie et inhibition des directions." Like much of Henry's aesthetic, many of the basic ideas and terminology for it come from contemporary biological or physiological research. Perhaps the most important of the terminology that Henry develops along these lines is that of "dynamogeny" and "inhibition," to which he devotes part 6 of the *Cercle chromatique*, pp. 138–64. The source of the idea of dynamogeny and inhibition is a certain M. Brown-Sequard. Actually, Henry mentions Brown-Sequard in "Une esthétique scientifique," p. 446, but the idea is not fully developed until the *Cercle chromatique*. For Henry, the idea or principle of dynamogeny and inhibition is universally applicable; this is so because there is a universal uniformity of structure or organic principle, the circle/cycle to which there has already been an allusion. An individual, an organ, a tissue, or a cell are all subject to the same laws or modes of behavior and interaction in terms of structure, energy, action, and motion.

Chapter Six

cycle moving dynamogenously from left to right and from low to high. This dynamogenously continuous experience is rare, most commonly our experience of sense reality is discontinuous. Each sensation is in the nature of a "stop"[12] within a given cycle, and the distinction between sensations is by way of *contrast,* which is the next basic principle upon which Henry elaborates:

> We have seen that there is no sensation without an arrest of movement and, by consequence, without virtual movement in an inverse direction. Every stop implies a virtual direction in a contrary sense. When the directions differ to a maximum or a minimum of perception, there is a stop on the cycle; this difference is the function of *contrast.*[13]

In addition, it can be said that contrast is either successive or simultaneous, though in actuality the successive actions of a living being are always virtually simultaneous.[14] That is, given two opposed directions simultaneously perceived, they are resolved into a new direction. Furthermore, Henry states two propositions relating to contrast of direction: first, *that every direction evokes its complementary;* secondly, given the meeting of two opposing directions, *every direction evokes the complementary of the other.*[15] Finally, a change of direction simultaneously perceived will be less than one successively perceived.[16]

Naturally, throughout his discussion on the phenomena of contrast Henry has recourse to various mathematical proofs of his ideas, including the relation of contrast to fundamental algorithms, an idea derived from *La Philosophie des mathé-*

12. Henry uses the word "arrêt," which I have variously translated as "stop" or "arrest."

13. *Cercle chromatique,* p. 24.

14. Ibid.

15. Ibid., p. 26.

16. Ibid., p. 27.

The Dynamist of Art

matiques by the curious transcendentalist Wronski.[17] Succession and simultaneity are seen as the two ways in which the unity may achieve its realization.[18] Finding that his own research correlates with that of Marey, Henry concludes that the number 12 represents the minimum and the maximum of divisions in which the unity can be realized in terms of the capacity of the two contrasts, successive or simultaneous. That is to say, following Wundt's investigations, twelve simple representations are the maximum extent of consciousness for maintaining relatively simple and successive representations. Henry concludes that consciousness is a "subjective function corresponding to the integral exercise of contrast."[19] The flow of mind, the psychocinematic continuum, is seen as a continual succession of contrasts of basic directions which in turn are perpetually and simultaneously evoking their complementaries or the complementaries of the directions with which they come in contact. In this complex process—the psychomathematics of the unconscious—consciousness is but a derivative, and illusions, optical or otherwise, are a commonplace, since rarely is one aware or conscious of the exact nature of the totality of directions to which the psychosensory nature is continually subject and with which it is interacting in the most unconscious of ways. It was one of Henry's social aims to utilize his mathematics of the unconscious in order to correct what he thought were

17. See chapter 5, n. 17. To the idea of succession belongs the fundamental algorithm of addition—"sommation"—and to the phenomena of simultaneity belongs multiplication (*Cercle chromatique*, pp. 29ff).
18. The unity, of Henry's Pythagorean assumption of universal interrelatedness, contains both the potential and the actual.
19. *Cercle chromatique*, p. 33. Henry's method is not easy to grasp. Everything must be considered as being measured on a circle or, more precisely, on the circumference of the circle. From a simultaneous point of view two directions will be contrasted to the minimum when the distance between them is $\frac{1}{2}$ the circumference; the maximum will be $\frac{1}{4}$. Minimum successive contrast is $\frac{1}{6}$, maximum is $\frac{1}{3}$. Thus the number 12 is at the same time the product of the minimum and the maximum of both kinds of contrast.

the various common illusions to which the psychosensory apparatus is subject and which is an aspect of the general social malaise. He speaks of constructing a dynamometric scale to this end.[20]

To continue with the fundamentals of Henry's aesthetic, given the phenomena of contrast, particularly that of successive contrast which occurs as a function of discontinuous cycles, one must then consider the larger whole, the functions of the cycles themselves, which can be reduced to the component aspects of rhythm and measure.

> We have seen how each variation of work of the living being is represented by a change of direction or, to put it otherwise, by a section of the circumference of a circle. What are the changes of dynamogenous direction? This is the problem of rhythm. In a given direction, which are the numbers of the dynamogenous points of arrest? This is the problem of measure.[21]

Again, the main reason for working out the mathematical basis for rhythmic figures is for the betterment of the psychosocial environment. Henry experiments with subjects in states of rest and fatigue in order to determine to which rhythms each of the corresponding states of consciousness is most responsive.

20. Ibid., p. 44. Was the *Échelles dynamométriques* ever published? We have been unable to locate it, though it is advertised on the back of the *Cercle chromatique*. The function of the *Échelles dynamométriques* was to permit "the rigorous proportioning of the state of energy of the subject," and was to include an introduction on "Pathogenie."

21. *Cercle chromatique*, p. 45. Discontinuous actions are those in which the force tends to the left; in continuous actions the force tends to the right; the complementary actions of discontinuous actions tend to be retarded. Below are two figures, representing figures 1 and 5 from the *Cercle chromatique*, and illustrating the various directions as complementary to one another.

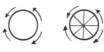

The Dynamist of Art

Fatigued, the subject will prefer inhibitory changes of directions expressed by the numbers 9, 11, 13; normal, he will prefer inhibitory changes of directions expressed by the numbers 6, 8, 10, 12.[22]

Henry finds that his theories are borne out by the experiments of Marey on the influence of rhythm on the speed of progression. In Marey's studies the curve of speed of progression corresponds to the rhythmic numbers 48, 51, 60, 64, 68, 80, 85.[23] Therefore, the curve proves that the speed of progression varies in nature with the function of the rhythm. From this Henry concludes that such curves can be drawn up to determine scales of dynamogeny and inhibition, again with the end of creating precise psychic effects or states of consciousness.

> Directly related to the problem of rhythm is that of measure. We have seen that the unit of measure is determined by a stop; as the living being is incapable of describing a straight line, he will consider the interval between two stops as a direction determining, within one direction or the other on the circumference, a section which corresponds to the minimum of a simultaneous contrast, that is ½, or to the minimum of successive contrast, ⅙: the unit of measure corresponds then to a cycle of equal diameter to this unity or double this unity; n points of arrest correspond to n cycles which are finally resolved in n sections of the great cycle, this

22. Ibid., pp. 46–47. Henry touched upon this problem later in one of his "À travers les sciences et l'industrie," articles, *Revue blanche* 7 (1894): 171–77, in discussing *La fatigue intellectuelle et physique* by M. Mosso. Henry concludes this article: "It will be a merit of M. Mosso to have posed and studied experimentally some of these questions which are of lively interest to all those who work, as well as to those who do nothing, and of which the importance will only increase all the more, the more one is convinced that philosophical sophisms, scientific errors, and aesthetic decadence (?) are nothing other than cerebral troubles, more or less collective."

23. *Cercle chromatique*, pp. 47–50. Henry bases himself on Marey's chronophotographs of running figures.

section having to be rhythmic. If the stops are unequally distant, the unit of measure will naturally be the smallest interval. The true unit would be the minimum perceptible; but this minimum being variable, because the living being tends to adopt by preference a unit relatively fixed, each time the common divider will be that much smaller. In general there will be measure if the final result yields, according to the appropriate direction, sums or differences of a rhythmic number.[24]

What this describes is the complexity of consciousness which is commonly taken for granted. In any case it is Henry's intention to determine those relations and proportions which are most dynamogenous and thus most life-enhancing.

A proportion is as dynamogenic as the fundamental algorithms of multiplication or addition, corresponding to succession and to simultaneity or their inverse aspects, and can be found implied in its terms. The two proportions which present this character are evidently of the form: $a/b = b/(a + b)$ known under the name of the *golden section,* and of the form $a/c = (a - b)/(b - c)$ called *harmonic* by the Greeks.[25]

Another premise which is basic to Henry's aesthetic is that there are two modes of action:

The mode of continuous action, characterized by the heightening of powers, or the inverse; the forms of contrast which mark the degree of continuity of these operations, play the role of exponents. The second is the mode of discontinuous action which becomes continuous according to whether the intervals are rhythmic and

24. Ibid., p. 50. A key passage. Of note is the idea that "the true unit would be the minimum perceptible; but this minimum being variable, *because the living being tends to adopt by preference a unit relatively fixed,* each time the common divider will be that much smaller." Herein, of course, lies the whole problem, the "relatively fixed units" which the individual tends to adopt being the source of all conflict and illusion since the adopted relatively fixed unit will then tend to be more and more at variance with the actuality of what is perceived.

25. Ibid., p. 52.

the numbers of the stops measued; this mode of action is characterized by the sums and their inverses.[26]

Henry then addresses himself to the problem of determining the mode of action which is absolutely discontinuous. Following Fechner, he considers the elementary sensation as a stop represented by the number e: the logarithms mark the degrees of continuity of a quantity of elementary arrests; the sensation corresponds to the natural logarithm of excitation.[27] However, this is only a gross approximation of the way things are, a criticism made by Bergson as well.[28] What is not considered in the Fechnerian formulation, which is primarily concerned with measuring the magnitude of sensation, is the character of the sensation or movement. Here Henry and Bergson are in accord, and it is to determine not only the magnitude, but the essential subjective character of sensation, that Henry addresses his experimental and mathematical aesthetic.

In summing up, the psychic functions being considered as virtual movements, and perception as a virtual realization of the object, the laws of perception are the forms imposed upon our representations by the modes of action of the living being. The relations by which phenomena are considered depend on the modes in which they are virtually realized and the mathematical operations correlative to these modes functioning in time. The agreeable or disagreeable action of living beings is nothing more than the continuity or discontinuity by which they realize themselves.[29]

26. Ibid., pp. 52ff. Like dynamogeny and inhibition, continuity and discontinuity are basic terminological concepts with Henry. Later in the *Cercle chromatique*, p. 162, Henry states, "It is to these double reactions of continuity and discontinuity that all scientific facts must be related, be they the subjective determinations which constitute mathematics, or the objective determinations which are the object of the natural sciences."
27. Ibid., pp. 53–54.
28. Ibid. See above, chapter 2, n. 16.
29. Ibid., pp. 54–55. A basic statement of Henry's thought.

Chapter Six

For the sake of clarification, let me recapitulate. What Henry describes in the first part of the *Cercle chromatique* is a general theory of interrelatedness and the laws which pertain to it: a general law of psychomotor reactions. Universal interrelations—the unity—is not a stasis but, according to the dynamics of Henry's thought, an indefinitively evolutive principle. The laws by which this unity functions are all of an essentially dynamic nature; beginning with the fundamental reality of direction, there follow the principles of dynamogeny and inhibition, successive and simultaneous contrast, and rhythm and measure with their concomitant aspects of cycles of continuity and discontinuity. The fundamental subjective or psychic reactions corresponding to the essentially positive/negative flux are pleasure and pain; on the one hand there is pleasure, continuity, and dynamogeny, and on the other pain, discontinuity, and inhibition. Consciousness of the functioning of the cosmic polarities and the dynamic process which they engender calls into play a moral/aesthetic imperative: that of seeing to it that the creation of ever more dynamogenous states of consciousness becomes the prevailing mode of action. In this way evolution, the ever greater expansion of consciousness, is fulfilled or realized.

It is precisely by the equation of inherently aesthetic reactions—agreeable/disagreeable, pleasurable/painful—to cosmic principles that Henry's bio-psycho-mathematical formulation of a theory of universal interrelatedness is also a fundamental system of aesthetics.

Henry applies the principles of his general theory to the elementary visual and auditory sensations, not in order to make any new hypotheses with regard to the structure and nature of the sense organs, but rather, given the already inherently dynamogenous or inhibitory structure of the senses, to understand how any given "form" tends to dynamogenize or inhibit us.[30] This is done with the obligatory intention of giving artists and society in general a basis for self-ameliora-

30. Ibid., p. 56.

114

tion through aesthetic means by indicating the dynamogenous principles by which such an end can be achieved. This evolutionary moral/aesthetic imperative is a basic feature of the psychophysical aesthetic created by Henry.

Henry's consideration of the visual sensation begins with the theory of directions.

> Visual sensation is projected in space; the representation of space as being continuous is projected on a cycle oriented within from left to right. But sensation is an arrest, thus the visual sensation is projected on a cycle oriented from right to left; it is discontinuous. The visual functions are decomposed according to their order of complexity, into sensation of light, sensation of color, sensation of form.[31]

Aesthetically, the problem is which directions to assign to these functions. Following the principles already elaborated with regard to cyclical directions, light is the primary visual sensation; accordingly it is projected mentally to the left, though the left eye is probably no more sensitive to light than the right. Corresponding to the sensations of light is a maximum of "elementary work."[32] As Henry points out, it is common sense that an eye reposing in darkness enjoys a light sensitivity far superior to an active eye; this is because when the eye which has been resting in darkness is exposed to the light a maximum of elementary work is required on the part of the entire retina to make the proper response. Slowly the eye makes its adjustments; like the prism, the eye decomposes light into color, creating a complex of psychophysical differentiations. But whereas light is a cyclical function that

31. Ibid., p. 57. Henry's basic formulation, of course, recalls Laforgue's essay on the "Impressionist Eye," and also Geroult's article, "Formes, couleurs, mouvements" (see above, chapter 4, n. 19). The decomposition of the visual sensation into light, color, and form is a fundamental idea of Henry's, and one he elaborates in an article entitled, "La lumière, la couleur et la forme," published in 1922 by Courbusier and Ozenfent in *L'esprit nouveau* (1921), pp. 605–23, 729–36, 948–58, 1068–75.

32. *Cercle chromatique,* pp. 58–59.

goes from left to right, the color function generally proceeds from right to left; the work of the eye increases in complexity but decreases in intensity. This is an aspect of right to left discontinuity. The next problem is assigning the directions corresponding to the different colors: this is done in the *Cercle chromatique,* the instrument or application of principles which Henry intended to offer as a "guide" for fulfilling the moral/aesthetic imperative of evolution, that is, the creation of dynamogenous states of consciousness.

The actual chromatic circle which Henry had engraved by a M. Rapine and published by a M. Chardon is essentially a corrected version of Chevreul's color wheel,[33] at least in its most superficial aspects. Spectral colors are dynamogenous and their sum is white; pigment colors are inhibitory and their sum is black. Black and white, the ultimately dynamogenous and inhibitory visual sensations, also correspond to the directions of continuity and discontinuity, left to right and right to left. The colors are then assigned directions according to their dynamogenous or inhibitory character. Red, "being the most dynamogenous because it sustains the most intense arrests of movement is assigned the direction from low to high"[34]—straight up, as it were. Blue is assigned the direction from right to left because of its essentially inhibitory character; yellow, from left to right. To the three primary colors correspond the three primary directions, and as each direction evokes its complementary, so does each color. This is the basic idea of Chevreul's simultaneous contrast which Henry obviously amplifies and expands, though with Henry the simultaneity of directions precedes that of colors, at least

33. E. Chevreul's chromatic circle was published again in *De la loi du contraste simultané des couleurs* (Paris, 1886). Chevreul's principle of simultaneous contrast is the most important idea Henry derives from the older scientist. With Henry the idea is elevated to a general psychic principle: all the senses experience simultaneous contrast, and to a very great degree what is called reality is much in the nature of an afterimage.
34. *Cercle chromatique,* p. 64.

in terms of general considerations. It is also well to recall that Laforgue voiced the same basic idea of light, color, and form in his article in impressionism and that, like Laforgue, who based himself in part on Hartmann and Helmholtz, Henry's theory is something of a synthesis of Chevreul and Goethe. In his *Farbenlehre*, Goethe emphasizes the subjective positive or negative nature of the various colors in much the same manner as Henry refers to the inherent dynamogeny or inhibition of colors.[35] Also with special reference to the manner or technique of the impressionist or neo-impressionist painters, Henry states that the eight pigmentary tones whose sum is black, and the six spectral tones whose sum is white, do not exclude each other but complete each other and answer to different points of view.[36] Then follows a curious illustration:

> *The Chromatic Circle* is theoretically constructed: the rational if not practical realization of it would be a resin cake of as great a radius as possible on which would be projected the ponderable proportions of the colored powders necessitated by the degradation of lights and of tints, assuring within perceptible limits the continuity of the sensation in surfaces and weights.[37]

Under the topic of direction with regard to visual sensation, Henry also discusses the continuity of white, the phenomena of irradiation, and various other factors pertaining directly to the sensation of light and its decomposition into colors, which further involves Henry in the continuity and discontinuity of clarity and visual acuity as well as the order

35. Goethe's *Farbenlehre* was published in 1817, largely as a rebuke to Newton's theory of prismatic colors, and as such is disreputably unscientific. Goethe's theory, on the other hand, has the merit of positing the *subjective* nature of color, that is, color as a psychological phenomenon rather than a merely physical one.
36. *Cercle chromatique*, p. 67. Nowhere does Henry seem to favor any one particular school or style.
37. Ibid.

in which the various spectral colors are productive of fatigue. Here again, much of what Henry says can be reduced to the basic principle of dynamogeny/inhibition and the theory of directions.

Following his general schema, Henry then proceeds to a discussion of contrast in the visual sensation. "Each light evokes its complementary, and in an ensemble of lights each evokes the complementary of the other."[38] The same, of course, is said of colors.[39] In keeping with the theory of directions, the sensation of color, like all sensations, is the realization of a change of direction.[40] Important to keep in mind is the essentially dynamic quality which Henry's correlation of direction and color yields, for the concept of direction is a psychophysical one involving an optical shift as well as a psychic one. It is this aspect of Henry's color theory which became so attractive to Delaunay, the synchromists, and Kupka in the post-cubist period, and which is similar to the theories put forward by Kandinsky in *On the Spiritual in Art.*[41]

Following various considerations on pigmentary and opti-

38. Ibid., p. 80.
39. Ibid., p. 82.
40. Ibid., p. 95.
41. With regard to art history, this area of Henry's influence has yet to be properly researched and assessed. See Herschel B. Chipp, "Orphism and Color Theory," *Art Bulletin* 40 (1958):57–58, who touches on Henry's influence and who interprets his theory as "purely" scientific and nonsymbolic (though Chipp does refer to Henry as a "poet in the circle of the Symbolists"). See also W. Kandinsky, *On the Spiritual in Art* (New York, 1946), pp. 43ff. Indeed, if Kandinsky does not evoke Henry, he certainly brings to mind Laforgue in such a passage as this: "Generally speaking, color directly influences the soul. Color is the keyboard, the eyes are the hammers, the soul is the piano with many strings. The artist is the hand that plays, touching one key or another purposively, to cause vibrations in the soul" (p. 45). Laforgue, of course, also developed a "keyboard" idea (see above, chapter 4). And although Kandinsky is considered by Chipp as "emotional" and generally adverse to scientific interpretation of color and form, Kandinsky proclaims that "The final abstract expression of every art is number (Ibid., p. 73)." See also chapter 8 below.

The Dynamist of Art

cal mixture as well as the application of the theory of directions and chromatic contrast to vegetal forms,[42] Henry discusses the application of rhythm and measure to the visual sensation. Here he works out his fundamental idea on the harmony of forms and the harmony of colors.[43] The basic consideration comes from Helmholtz, who puts forth the idea of the movements of the eyes as being comparable to the functions of the compass. Because of the circular form of the eye, its movements can be described in terms of cycles, and the cycles therefore can be rhythmically coordinated, thus inducing the desired dynamogenous state of consciousness. This is done by adjusting *form,* which, according to Henry, is a compendium of directions, so that the form is a harmony of directions productive of a rhythmic number and thus visually perceived as a function for a rhythmic cycle. This is the harmony of forms. The same method applies to color which, as we have seen, is also a function of the theory of directions.

To give artists, art historians, industrial designers, and artisans and workers in general an index, as it were, for the rectification and harmonizing of all forms, Henry created in conjunction with the *Cercle chromatique* the *Rapporteur esthétique,* in which essentially the same ideas are expressed with regard to the functions of light, color, and form. That is, in a great cycle, light functions from left to right; color, depending on whether it is spectral or pigmentary, left to right or right to left but tending to go down; and form from right to left but going up. With regard to the necessity of creating rhythmic forms, Henry again states the moral/aesthetic imperative by pointing out that rhythm is naturally conducive

---

42. *Cercle chromatique,* p. 100. Again, in order to make his theories as universal as possible, Henry refers to experimentation with primary biological and, in this case, even zoological phenomena to prove that all of life participates and responds in the same basic ways to the equally universal phenomena of light and color.

43. Ibid., pp. 101ff.

to health and lack of rhythm to a lack of health. Health corresponds to dynamogenous states, illness to inhibitory ones. Henry concludes that the method of the *Rapporteur esthétique,* and by extension of his aesthetic in general, is to be applied to all forms, archaeological or present-day. He adds:

> But we will not pretend that I wish to substitute for the creation of the artist the mechanism of an instrument . . . the artist is only an eye, an ear, a nervous system normally organized and developed: he feels a rhythm, and because he feels it, because the idea is a virtual realization, he produces it exteriorly. He feels and produces it well, the more normal and harmonious the milieu. There are no schools. But it is the brilliant social states, such as Greece or the Renaissance, which produce the great periods of art. Reciprocally, to help the normal development of art is to favor as much the still distant realization of our destiny—the creation of universal harmony.[44]

Pursuing the aim of helping to create a state of more universal harmony, Henry published in 1891 *Harmonie de formes et de couleurs,* and *L'Education du sens des formes,* with plates by Paul Signac. This last work again deals with a basic instruction on the harmony of lights, colors, and forms derived from the theory of directions, dynamogeny/inhibition, contrast and rhythm and measure. It was published under the auspices of the Ministry of Commerce, Industry, and the Colonies, with the view of introducing these studies into the technical schools. Henry himself applied his method archaeologically,[45] in analyzing the formal calculations made from a Knidian amphora.

And finally, again with the aid of Paul Signac, Henry re-

44. *Rapporteur esthétique,* p. 16.
45. *Application de nouveaux instruments de précision a l'archéologie* (Paris, 1890).

states his theory in "L'esthétique des formes" published in four parts in the *Revue blanche* (1894–95).[46]

Perhaps the most interesting idea put forth in this last-mentioned work is the "unconscious calculations of forms."[47] This is but a further expression of the idea of direction as a psychophysical reality. In actuality every sensory impression is accompanied by an *unconscious* calculation of directional change; the mind creates unconsciously what the senses experience. This is a formulation of the idea of the archetype, which can be defined as a form projected by the unconscious and endowed with certain powers of a psychic nature. Obviously the power of such forms is in proportion to how rhythmic and harmonious their essential structure is. As an example, Henry reproduces the archetypal form of an elegant cross with a detailed mathematical analysis of its structural elements which proves these elements to be uniquely rhythmic.[48] Such uniquely rhythmic figures naturally have a pro-

---

46. In addition to having "discovered" Henry for the neo-impressionists, Paul Signac is the one artist who actively collaborated with Henry, mostly by making designs according to Henry's calculations of rhythmic or nonrhythmic numbers. In addition, Signac executed a poster for Henry (see *Harmonies de formes et de couleurs*, pp. 59–60) where Henry describes a work in which "each letter is inscribed in my chromatic circle; only following the lines, the circle turns different angles by relation to its natural orientation." It is not at all clear whether this is the same poster that Signac did for the Théâtre Libre in 1888 and which carries the inscription in the lower right-hand corner "application du Cercle chromatique de Mr. Ch. Henry" and to which Fénéon devoted a short article in *La revue Indépendante* (October, 1888), pp. 137–38. It seems possible that Signac did two posters according to the *Cercle chromatique*. In addition to these various projects by Signac directly related to Henry, there is the *Portrait of Fénéon,* which I shall consider in the next chapter. Despite Signac's close association with Henry, Lövgren's assessment seems most just: "Signac's own writings and paintings show that he had, to a certain extent, become entangled in colour-technical problems and occasionally found it difficult to follow Henry on his way towards 'absolute beauty'" (*Modernism,* p. 71).

47. "L'esthétique des formes," 515ff.

48. Ibid., pp. 520–21.

found effect on the unconscious which then endows the figure with symbolic, archetypal, and psychic powers. Here is a glimpse of what Henry meant by a "symbolic calculus," as well as the significance of what he would have called dynamogenous forms. Far from creating the basis for an "abstract art" barren of reference to reality, as such art is commonly conceived,[49] Henry creates the aesthetic of an art which is profoundly symbolic and psychological in the sense of affecting the state of consciousness to the point of its alteration; this is not an art barren of all reference to reality, but one which is totally imbued with it. Here we can recall Henry's pronouncement made in 1891 concerning the "imminent advent" of a profoundly mystical art.[50]

But on the whole, Henry's aesthetic is couched in concise scientific terminology, and the essentials of it, as we have indicated, can all be found in the *Cercle chromatique*. In addition to stating a general theory of universal interrelatedness and the application of the laws pertaining to it to the visual sensation (as I have stated, the psychophysicist describes reality in terms of sense experience and not in terms of an abstract "matter"), Henry also applies these principles to the auditory sensation. As might be expected, the structure of the auditory experience is analogous to that of the visual; Henry's method of analysis only adds to the similarity in the basics of these two sensations. The similarity of sense functions is, of course, a formulation of the primary symbolist idea that all of the arts are analogous, borne out by the experience of synesthesia; being analogous, the arts ought to be combined

49. As example of what I indicate here, Robert L. Herbert in *Neo-Impressionism*, p. 23, defines "abstract" as " 'devoid of reference to the real world,' as we now use the term." To me this definition of abstract is the ultimate absurdity; that which is devoid of reference to the real world is nothing, since the real world is always a subjective definition anyway. This definition of abstract is the definition of the aesthetic "purist," who is ultimately anaesthetic.

50. See above, p. 27.

in order to create aesthetically the extremely pleasurable experience of synesthesia.[51] This, incidentally is a state which Henry describes as physiological white; just as white light is the synthesis or sum of the spectral colors, simultaneously perceived, so physiological white is the synthesis or sum of the chromatics of all the senses simultaneously perceived or experienced. It is altogether possible that this is a description of the mystical experience.[52]

In any case, though the sensations are analogous and can therefore be described and analyzed by the same principles —the theory of directions, and so on—the auditory sensation differs from the visual. The latter is:

> simultaneously triple—luminous, chromatic, schematic; the auditory sensation is simple. Complex, the visual unity would appear under the form of a great cycle of a discontinuous reaction from two sides. Simple, the auditory unity would appear under the form of a small continuous cycle. Thus each variation of excitation is marked first of all by a variation in the number of circumferences executed in order to be able to project the changes of direction of a relatively discontinuous cycle. The visual sensation is projected on a cycle oriented from right to left and tending upward; the auditory sensation is normally projected on a cycle oriented from left to right and tending upward, for the visual sensa-

---

51. See above, chapter 5, n. 35.

52. Henry indicates as much when in describing these states he refers to the famous Dervishes. Thus too, in a classic mystical text like the *Tibetan Book of the Dead,* ed. W. Y. Evans-Wentz (Oxford, 1927), the key liberating experience is marked by the vision of the "fundamental Clear light." This Clear light, or bright white light, which indicates the ultimate experience probably relates to the Laforgue/Henry idea that the purest experience of the eye is one of pure white undifferentiated light. Perhaps Henry's physiological white can be considered as both the primary experience and the final or ultimate experience, if, indeed, there is any real difference between these two; mystically speaking, there probably is not! See above, chapter 5, n. 15.

tion is the arrest of a representation in space . . . the auditory sensation is an instant of time.[53]

From this follows the difference in the conditions of dynamogeny. The dynamogeny of a color is correlative to its wave length and consequently inversely related to the number of vibrations in a unit of time. The dynamogeny of sound is correlative to the number of vibrations in a unit of time or to the number of instants considered simultaneously. Acute sounds would appear to be high and relatively dynamogenous, deep sounds low and inhibitory; these correspond to the directions of inner work, the psychic attributions as it were. As an instance of the general evolution of sensation and the corresponding progress in the psychic complexity of humanity, Henry makes note once again of the fact that the Greeks had the opposite association of sounds, that is, the direction of "high" was associated with "deep" sounds and "low" with the higher-pitched sounds. This would only seem natural because the Greeks, at least according to Henry, witnessed only the most objective character of their representations. The power of these exterior or objective representations—gestures, cries, and attitudes—is rigorously inverse to the complexity of interior representations. Presumably, progress is an increase in the understanding of the complexity of interior representations and inner work that go into one exterior form or symbol. Furthermore, it can be said that, as with visual representations, there is a symbolic calculus for the auditory as well as all the other senses; one can infer that

53. *Cercle chromatique*, p. 112. Below are reproduced three figures, representing figures 2, 3, and 10 from the *Cercle chromatique*, and illustrating the cycles referred to in this passage.

Continuity/   Discontinuity/   Triple Simultaneity
Dynamogeny   Inhibition   of Visual Sensation

The Dynamist of Art

there are symbolic or archetypal sounds as there are archetypal forms, sounds uniquely rhythmic which create in the
mind reactions of great psychic potency.[54]

In his discussion of music—the auditory sensation—Henry
displays a great range of knowledge extending from Pythagoras and Ptolemy to Wronski and Helmholtz. In addition,
Henry continually makes correspondences between aspects
of sound and vision by virtue of the mathematical analysis
which reveals the same *relationships* in terms of continuity
and discontinuity of experience in both the auditory and visual senses. In his analysis of the properties of the melodic
scale and the harmonic scale, Henry makes the further analogy that each scale, like the spectral or pigmentary colors of
the painters, presents a point of view, and that the melodic
scale can be compared to the pigmentary point of view of
the painters. Of course, the whole discussion is made with
reference to dynamogeny and inhibition, harmony and dissonance.

In some cases, Henry makes some most interesting infer-
ences. Given the theory of vibrations so essential to an understanding of the function of sound upon the auditory sense,
Henry sees no reason why this should not apply to the sense-

54. See above, chapter 3, n. 65, for a brief discussion of the important
implications of this idea. As we have mentioned earlier, the works of René
Ghil provide an interesting example of literary theories developed along
principles similar to those suggested by Henry: See René Ghil, *Traité du
verbe*, first published in 1886, and later amplified, in which Ghil develops
a theory of instrumentation based on "scientific" principles which is combined with a mystical evolutionary idea. Ghil, like many of his symbolist
contemporaries, was aware of the Vedas and the traditions of India. Thus
in a poem from the *Cantilènes* by Jean Moreas (1886) there is a reference
to Maya, "L'astucieuse et belle," to which Fénéon adds the comment that
in addition to being sonorous, with interlacing rhythms, there is in this
poem "a vocabulary of a mathematical precision" (Fénéon, *Oeuvres*, p.
221). And in an article on another writer, Charles Vignier, whom Fénéon
calls a "Poète français et psychophysicien" (*Oeuvres*, pp. 241ff.), there is
further evidence of a very great influence of psychophysics on the literary
symbolists. Naturally in this last mentioned article on Charles Vignier,
Fénéon calls attention to the theory of directions in the "fecund doctrine
of Charles Henry."

body in general. Just as different musical instruments give different forms of vibrations, so different media and materials can and must be exploited so that the senses will be properly enriched by as wide a spectrum of harmonic vibrations as possible. "In this is the major importance of techniques; it belongs to our century, so rich in industrial means, to reopen and enlarge infinitely the way of these superior harmonies which the refined aesthetic of the Greeks did not neglect."[55] On the other hand, Henry concludes his investigation of the auditory sensation with a statement on the inherent limitations of sense experience:

> But there is an abyss between the complex rhythms which become realizable in time and the number which are unrealizable due to our natural mechanics. There is no more of a common measure for us between sorrow and pleasure than between nothingness and existence.[56]

What Henry seems to be paraphrasing here is the truth of the saying that heard melodies are sweet, but those unheard are sweeter by far. But this again draws attention to the fact that what Henry presents, however mathematical and erudite, is a transcendental aesthetic: a call for the creation of a common measure between nothingness and being.

Henry devotes the last part of the *Cercle chromatique* to a detailed discussion of the principle of dynamogeny and inhibition, continuity and discontinuity, a principle which is amazingly flexible and which can be applied to all excitants: electricity, heat, weight, odor, taste, and so on.[57] In language for instance, Henry sees in vowels a continuous mode of re-

55. *Cercle chromatique*, p. 135.
56. Ibid., p. 137.
57. Ibid., pp. 138ff. On p. 149, Henry again relates the activities of individual organisms, in this case the act of love, to the magnetic intensity of the planet, suggesting a more cosmic reorientation of our various activities; he considers how it is now well known that the body responds to electrical impulses, and that the cells of the brain in particular are centers of intense electrical activity. In his speculations on the matter of electromagnetic orientation, Henry again invites comparison with Edwin Babbitt.

action, in consonants a discontinuous one; from this, obviously, an aesthetic science of language could be formulated. In fact, to follow Henry's thesis to its conclusion, all of life ought to be aesthetically regulated in such a way that every last gesture of life itself would be an aesthetic expression: the final condition of universal harmony which Henry envisions is a "recovery" of the "ritual disposition," that disposition in which every action (direction) is invested with cosmic significance.[58] To understand the dynamogenous and inhibitory functions of all our actions and sensations, that is, to become conscious of them through heightened aesthetic awareness, is to become conscious of what is called in psychology the law of the association of ideas, which, as Henry points out, is no different from the functions of contrast, rhythm, and measure without which there can be no continuity of virtual movements which are called ideas.[59]

> The normal fact of the transformation of a sensation into an idea is a fact of successive contrast. In effect we have seen how all sensation corresponds to an arrest and every idea to a virtual movement which becomes real: for there is no arrest without (1) a direction in a certain sense (unconscious intuition), and (2) a direction in an inverse sense, which corresponds to the correlative reaction, idea. On the other hand, in hallucination, spontaneous or provoked (suggestion), it is the idea which is transformed into an unconscious intuition which leads to a sensation.[60]

This fact demonstrates the fluidity of the whole phenomenon of consciousness and, in the words of Brown-Sequard, shows that "hypnotism is only an effect and an ensemble of acts of inhibition and of dynamogeny."[61] For Henry even the most

58. The phrase "ritual disposition" is a Chinese one; see Mai-Mai Sze, *The Way of Chinese Painting* (New York, 1959), chapter 1, "The Concept of Tao."
59. *Cercle chromatique,* p. 141.
60. Ibid.
61. Ibid., p. 142.

complex psychic phenomena can be reduced to functions of the circle, for the phenomena of dynamogeny and inhibition as continuity and discontinuity, are themselves cyclical functions of a reciprocal nature. As a result of the reciprocal nature of all phenomena—interrelatedness—Henry envisions the following:

> the reality of a superior coordination of the virtual movements of individuals, just as the individual is a coordination of real movements of centers of an inferior order: the species then is quite really and not metaphorically an organism, but an organism of a virtual order, rhythmic or not, depending on whether the individuals are rhythmic or not. The problem of dynamogeny and inhibition is then posed for the species as it is for the individual. But for the species there will be no more virtual absolute rhythm unless it is able to realize all its numbers by a real coordination of individual centers. These centers will necessarily be obliged to be rhythmic, otherwise all coordination would be impossible. The development of the individual is as impossible without the development of the species as the development of the species is impossible without the development of the individual.[62]

From this Henry deduces his law of evolution: in rhythmic, dynamogenous actions is the evolutionary mechanism of life, because dynamogeny is naturally expansive.

> The conscious concordance of an exterior mode of action and a mode of representation constitutes the truth, and the development of the correlative power which gives us science is only a concrete manifestation of this harmony.
> From this, three facts: (1) the tendency of the species to transform a discontinuous mode of action into a continuous one, a tendency which can only be realized by a unity of action; (2) individual tendency towards

62. Ibid., pp. 143–44.

The Dynamist of Art

dynamogeny; (3) representation for the individual in his virtual cyclical functions of an infinity of changes of direction which, nonrhythmic for his unicentral mechanics, are actually realizable only by an intelligent coordination of centers. The result of this important consequence is that individuality tends to be collective, and that collectivity tends to be individual. The realization of this double end would be the age of absolute harmony; the complexity of the rhythm which sweeps the species along is the same in consequence for the individual.[63]

Such is the vision of Charles Henry, "dynamist of art." Though mathematically complex, in its essentials the aesthetic developed is simple and dynamic. Through a basic psychological/symbolical means, that of directions rhythmically ordered, art ought to be dynamogenized: indeed, art is a dynamogenous function. In the aesthetic/moral imperative of furthering evolution—progress if you will—Henry's aesthetic is akin to that of William Morris, or even of Gauguin, both of whom, like Henry, were instrumental in the creation of art nouveau as a profound cultural manifestation which exhibited a stylistic unity unknown to Europe since the Neoclassical style. Certainly art nouveau is a dynamogenous style, whose forms are self-developing and symbolic in the sense of appealing directly to the precognitive regions of consciousness. In Henry's words, it can be said that the essential characteristic of art nouveau is the extent to which the *rhyth-*

63. Ibid., pp. 147–48. As a predecessor, Henry evokes the name of Charles Fourier, an earlier nineteenth-century French scientist with an equally utopian disposition, but whose imagination, according to Henry, forgot the preliminary necessity of a "physiological evolution towards the normal, an evolution which will be the consequence of an industrial art, of a superior spiritual hygiene, and of the introduction of a motor as perfect as possible in the various industries so that aesthetic activity can be rendered attractive." Presumably, Henry has in mind a utopia in which the perfection of the machine is the liberation of man into a situation in which the practice and cultivation of what we call the arts is the sole or major aim of the race.

mic changes of directions of the representations create reactions correspondingly rhythmic, continuous, and dynamogenous. In art nouveau it is the dynamic direction of line which is of the essence.

This is a general conclusion that can be reached about the influence of Henry's aesthetic; this kind of effect will also be seen in the post-Cubist painters—the Delaunays, Kupka, Kandinsky, and the synchromists, all of whose art might best be categorized as dynamogenously oriented. As an example of a more immediate effect of Henry's aesthetic, the idiosyncratic portrait of Fénéon by Signac will now be analyzed.

7
Paul Signac's
Against the Enamel of a Background Rhythmic with Beats and Angles, Tones and Colors. Portrait of M. Félix Fénéon in 1890, Opus 217

S PEAKING of music in his *Introduction à une esthétique scientifique,* Charles Henry takes into account the idea of "continual autogenesis,"[1] an intuitive concept which is the energy source and content of arabesque—musical as well as visual. By arabesque one can understand any "decorative" motif: often intricate, repetitive, self-reproductive, and, ideally, self-mutative. This dynamically creative, or procreative, energy principle is evident in much of so-called primitive art, often in the variant form of the meander and zig-zag, as well as being a basic factor on the phase of Western art that we call art nouveau. As such, continual autogenesis is a universal principle, transcultural and embracing all media, for it is an organic or natural principle. One may even say that reality itself is a process of continual autogenesis. When Henry's ideas were first published and heard, "au temps du symbolisme," the analogy between painting and music offered by the concept of continual autogenesis easily took root in certain receptive minds.

An aspect of this idea—continual autogenesis—can be seen in the painting by Signac with the elaborate and humorous title, *Against the Enamel of a Background Rhythmic with Beats and Angles, Tones and Colors, Portrait of M. Félix Fé-*

1. See above, chapter 5, n. 37.

Chapter Seven

néon in 1890, Opus 217.[2] Signac at the time was, of course, a
disciple of Henry, collaborating as a draughtsman with the
experimental psychologist in various works, notably the
Cercle chromatique, the *Rapporteur esthétique,* and "L'esthétique des formes." All these works are of a highly abstract
and mathematical nature, for it was Henry's idea, quite simply, that there is a simultaneous one-to-one relationship between outer stimulus and psychic or perceptual reaction
which can be mathematically calculated. What is interesting
and most pertinent in Henry's aesthetic is that it deals solely
with the correspondence of psychic experience to sensory
experience. Art is understood as a medium affecting the relation between sense and psyche; visually, this is done with
color and line. Accordingly the way is opened for an understanding that takes place at a nonverbal or, more appropriately, a psychic level: knowledge or understanding is an identification of sensory and psychic transmissions.

In view of this it is not surprising that Paul Signac should
apotheosize the critic/champion of neo-impressionism, Félix
Fénéon, in a painting which, with its cyclical flow of arabesque, stars, and sundry color patterns is also an attempted
compendium of Henry's ideas visually translated. Such a
painting is obviously "unique," representing as it does a kind
of self-conscious tribute to itself: in one sense a brilliant example of feedback, it is also the "final" work of neo-impres-

2. The painting, long in the collection of Félix Fénéon, is now in a private collection in New York. For its history, see *Signac* (Paris: Musée du
Louvre), catalogue to the Signac exhibition held December, 1963, to February, 1964; see also Herbert, *Neo-Impressionism,* pp. 140–41, in which
the painting is described as a "sport amidst the flora of neo-impressionism
. . . the background is a direct evocation of Charles Henry." But little further reference is made to *how* the background is an evocation of Charles
Henry; on the other hand the background is compared to a painting by
Rossetti, *Dantis Amore,* though this seems untenable and only coincidental. Furthermore, in the Herbert text Fénéon is described as holding a
"decadent lily," though there is no reason to believe this, especially since
the cyclamen is a flower *symbolically* much more in keeping with the
content of the painting as well as Henry's philosophy, with its emphasis
on *cycles.*

Signac's Portrait of Fénéon

sionism, first exhibited in March, 1891, just after the death of Seurat. Certainly no other neo-impressionist work carries further the basic ideas of the movement, taking them to so final an "abstract" or "decorative" level. Seurat's *La Cirque*, is a beautiful example of the process of reduction almost to the point of caricature, as is the depiction of Fénéon by Signac, but beyond that we are dealing with two different ideas entirely.

Although it is evident that there is a certain whimsey to this work, since the critic Fénéon, a man of driest wit, was viewed, with goatee and top hat, as a kind of Uncle Sam, there is more than passing allusion to the character of this symbolist mystifier profiled in Signac's painting. Even the title, *Against the Enamel of a Background. . . .* , suggests Fénéon's influence or character. There is no "enamel" but rather the use of the word "enamel" is a typical symbolist device: to suggest or evoke a hard, polished, decorative, jewelled or even synthetic surface, totally "unreal." After all, in his biography of Signac, also published in 1890, at the time Signac was doing his portrait, Fénéon did indicate that by order of the Emerald Archetype Tetrarch Signac would be promised the title of "official landscapist of the Esoteric White Islands."[3] In the simplest sense, Signac's opus 217 can be seen as a portrait in profile against a completely decorative background. However, since Signac worked so closely with Henry, and since Henry's thought is so systematic, as was Signac's, at least at the time the portrait was painted, the "enamel background" deserves more attention than it has thus far been given, for certainly it is not just an arbitrary "background." Signac, following Henry, and in the wake of Richard Wagner, knew that painting and music were analogous, that painting should aspire to what one may call the flowing nonspecificity of music, for at root both arts are engendered and activated by the same principle, continual autogenesis. This is where Seurat's

3. Félix Fénéon, "La peinture optique: Paul Signac," first published in 1890, re-published in *Au delà de l'impressionnisme* (Paris, 1966), p. 120.

work left off in 1891, and this is what the portrait of Fénéon is finally about. From about 1886 to the early 1890s Signac labelled all of his works with opus numbers, but it is only in the *Portrait of Fénéon* that Signac attempts a real break with the idea of painting as representation. It is in the background of this painting that Signac's understanding of Henry is revealed as visual music.

The ground of opus 217 is basically an example of the process of continual autogenesis. There is a center-point (though not the actual pictorial center) from which all flows, or into which all flows—most probably both. The ground is divided into eight parts, the whole of which together could extend or expand indefinitely. In this there is a very strong kinetic sensation like that of a pinwheel in motion. This, of course, is a *perceptual* phenomenon which accentuates the idea of continual autogenesis—the inexhaustible energy flow which animates the reality of forms. At this point what has been described is already a realm of art or experience quite distinct from that of the representational portrait: the "background" of this painting is an essay in pure visual perception, at the very least. The figure of Fénéon, on the other hand, is understood first of all at the semantic level of cognition, literally as a representation of some *body*. Significantly, Fénéon, the literary symbolist, holds in his right hand a symbol, the cyclamen flower, which is the representational key or link to the enamel ground which is executed as a cycle perpetually in motion. There is here an antithesis of the static —the angular representation of Fénéon—and the dynamic— the "enamel" cycle of visual perception. This may also be something of a reference to Henry's concept of universal polarity: the "inhibitory," or the angular Fénéon, and the "dynamogenic," or the ground.[4]

4. As I have indicated in the previous chapter, dynamogeny and inhibition are two absolutely key ideas in the work of Henry. For Fénéon, Henry's central idea could be summed up as the theory of dynamogeny; thus, in an article on Henry's publication of *Oeuvres et Correspondances*

Signac's Portrait of Fénéon

Furthermore, each of the areas of the enamel cycle has a separate design and/or color idea which also contributes to the sense of infinite expansion. Beginning with the upper left, there is a purple and yellow arabesque, probably a specific reference to the idea of continual autogenesis as arabesque already mentioned. Then follow two areas of alternating bands of color: blue and orange, and yellow and violet, each pair being a complementary contrast executed, as is the entire surface of the painting, in the uniform neo-impressionist manner of the divided tone for optical mixture. The fourth area contains a number of yellow "planetary" emblems on a violet ground. The fifth band is a series of yellow five-pointed stars on a blue ground, followed by a flow-area of pale blue flower-petal forms, probably a reference to the cyclamen which Fénéon holds. The seventh area is a typical neo-impressionist color exercise, primarily blue intermingled with its complementary, orange, and going from almost white at the center to darkest and most intense tonality at the outer edge—the effect is like that of a vibratory flow.[5] The final area is red and its complementary, green, patterned so that the lightest hues are juxtaposed where the two colors meet and darkest where they are farthest apart. Within this area, red moves "up," green moves "down." In connection with this particular, it should be noted that in Henry's *Aesthetic of*

---

inédites de d'Alembert, Fénéon, commenting on the various aesthetic theories of d'Alembert and Rameau, states that "These theories, like those of today, for example, that of Helmholtz, were purely objective, and therefore, vain. It will belong to the imminent theory of dynamogeny of Charles Henry to reduce consonance, dissonance, melody, harmony, modes to the absolutely general subjective functions of contrast, rhythm, and measure" (Fénéon, *Oeuvres,* pp. 278–81).

5. The gradation effect is also reminiscent of the gradation of the chromatic circle in which the center, being representative of the optical mixture of the prismatic colors, is white. Of course the white center is also a symbolic white, with reference to Henry's idea of "physiological white" —the purity of the experience of the center of being—which is the synesthetic effect of total simultaneous perception. That this should be a vibratory flow is natural.

Chapter Seven

Forms, on which Signac was collaborating in the early 1890s, the psychophysicist states that the direction of red is up and from left to right, whereas green is down and from right to left, as in this painting.[6]

Quite evidently, the ground of the Fénéon portrait is a continuity of energy areas moving in a cyclical manner from left to right—clockwise. This is in exact correspondence with Henry's *Rapporteur esthétique,* where, after formulating once again his basic idea that the aesthetic problem is both psychological and formal, a matter of psychic continuity or discontinuity corresponding through process of perception to experiences of pleasure or pain, Henry posits the idea that the inner psychic motion can be scientifically calculated. The psychophysiologist states that it is possible to create a "direct symbolical calculus" based on the notion that there is a corresponding psychic motion or direction to every external stimulus.[7] In speaking of the sensation of form, Henry conceives of reality in terms of cycles of perception. He says that the cycle of continuous movement—the projection of space —goes from left to right. The cycle of discontinuous movement—the projection of time—goes from right to left. According to Henry, visual sensation is related to the cycle of discontinuous motion, because forms are composed of series of discontinuous directions. On the other hand, the visual sensation is first of all a matter of experiencing light; then follows the experience of color; and finally, increasing in complexity, comes the experience of form. The primal sensation of light is continuous—there are no "stops" or changes

6. *Revue blanche* 7 (1895):308–22, though the idea is treated as early as "Une esthétique scientifique" in 1885, as well as in the *Cercle chromatique* where Henry states that red is the most dynamogenous color, and therefore, its direction is as it is in this section of the painting.

7. *Rapporteur esthétique,* p. 6. Also with regard to the general circular motion of the ground of this painting, it is well to keep in mind Henry's idea that "from the point of view of consciousness, the form of the movements of expression is circular" (*Sur la dynamogenie et l'inhibition* [Paris, 1889]).

of direction—while that of form is discontinuous. That is to say, forms are composed of a discontinuity of directions. The sensation of light, according to Henry, creates a psychic motion that goes from left to right, the sensation of form from right to left, corresponding to the cycles of continuous and discontinuous motion, respectively.[8]

In the painting, Signac has Fénéon facing left; he is a representational form as such, a totality of various discontinuous directions, whereas the ground of the painting is a definite cycle whose continuous perceptual direction is from left to right, the direction of light and the cycle of continuous motion. Signac has, by use of contrasting principles, given us the projection of a visual phenomenon in time—the representational form of Fénéon, an angular and rectilinear paradigm of Henry's concept of the discontinuity of form—and the projection of space, which is by nature continuously cyclical, therefore partaking of the same energy flow and psychic direction which characterizes the sensation of light, and which Signac has linked up with the idea of continual autogenesis.

At this point the whole idea of the enamel ground against which Fénéon is placed by Signac becomes cosmic in conception, for Signac, at least at this time, must have known from Henry that reality is a matter of subjective perception, that what is perceived is energy, a self-generating, vibratory activity which is finally inseparable from the psychic reactions it induces. As Henry later pointed out, this energy flow is as much a function of our being as it is a cosmic function—we are essentially biological resonators.[9] Further indication of the "cosmic" content besides the implication of infinity of the cyclical motion—the cycle or circle is the universal symbol of infinity or, rather, eternity—are Signac's inclusion of "planetary" and astral emblems, as well as the arabesque and flow of flower petals. Indeed, what is represented, in how-

8. See above, chapter 6, pp. 115–18.
9. This, of course is a key idea Henry develops in his later work, especially the already cited *Théorie du rayonnement*.

ever inarticulate and unconscious a manner, is an expression of the cosmic law in which everything is included or involved: the cycle of continuous motion—all light, all energy, planetary, astral, and organic forms are bound in one activity, one great celestial act, proceeding from and/or met in one center, as complete, simultaneous, and magical as if it were indeed the perception Saint Fénéon were having of the cyclamen which he extends in his right hand.

The extent to which Signac was aware in the *Portrait of Fénéon* of the cosmic content and implications of Henry's ideas was probably not profound, and maybe like Pissarro he saw no further point in such a "meaningless" use of arabesque and other decorative schemes.[10] On the other hand, such ideas bordering on the mystical or the occult were not uncommon with the symbolists, Signac's peers and friends, and it is difficult to think that Signac was not affected by such ideas. In fact, the idea of synthesis, so dear to the symbolists, finally comes down to a union of all factors, forms, and modes of knowing and experience; and the expression of this idea is clear in the enamel ground of the Fénéon painting, opus 217. Synthesis of the sort Signac attempted is not just an approximation of visual music, but a reformulation in paint of the cosmic law which one *knows* only at the most profound levels of psychic experience. In this regard, it is interesting that Signac has divided his cycle into eight parts, perhaps in relation to the idea of the octave, a musical as well as an occult concept, which itself comprises a complete cycle.[11]

10. C. Pissarro, *Lettres à son fils Lucien* (Paris, 1950), p. 222. If the *Portrait of Fénéon* appeared senseless to Pissarro, it should also be remembered that Seurat had to explain Henry's theories to Pissarro earlier in the mid-'80s and that by the time the *Portrait* was exhibited in 1891 Pissarro had fallen away from the theories adhered to by the neo-impressionists.

11. Particular attention is devoted to the idea of the octave in the system of Gurdjieff and Ouspensky. See especially P. D. Ouspensky, *In Search of the Miraculous* (New York, 1949), where the idea of the octave is very extensively developed in conjunction with the idea of the cyclical motion of activity in general; this idea is very close to that of Henry's. The system of Gurdjieff/Ouspensky is developed from basic Sufi ideas, and it is in-

Signac's Portrait of Fénéon

It is also fruitful to note in passing that the idea of a visual formulation of cosmic law with a definite center and geometrically composed—here a "pinwheel"—has its affinities not only with the "abstract" painting developed in the twentieth century, but with an earlier or more distant mode of "abstraction," the mandala, whose function is not pure aesthetic appreciation, but magical involvement: total psychic participation. Whether it was Signac's aim to create a work whose function was psychic involvement, we cannot say; but as an expression of ideas derived from Henry's psychology of perception, Signac's opus 217 can be seen as an experiment in this direction.

Indeed, neo-impressionism as it is commonly understood is only tangential to Henry's aesthetic as a whole. The significance of the *Portrait of Fénéon* is that it is truly an attempt at expressing the totality of Henry's thought, which by its nature must be expressed in other than merely representational forms. In this respect, the enamel ground is an elaborated representation of Henry's essential idea. This idea is his conception of the biopsychic norm which can be described as a circle and its center point. The extensions of the body are literally appendices to this norm.

The concept is a highly esoteric or mystical one, the circle naturally being considered the absolute symbol of perfection. From the pre-Socratics and Plato through the hermetic texts, down through Dante, Pascal, and the classical mathematicians, the circle or sphere is a magical figure. This is psychophysically stated in Henry's reduction of all phenomena

---

teresting to note with regard to the *Portrait of Fénéon,* with its eight-part cyclical, kaleidoscopic motion, that it is a typical Sufi practice to create vehicles—poetic, mythical, scientific, or whatever—that "are susceptible of another interpretation: a sort of demonstration analogous to a kaleidoscopic effect. And when Sufis draw diagrams for such purposes as these, imitators merely tend to copy them and use them at their own level of understanding" (Shah, *Sufi Ideas,* p. 20). Shah also comments on this matter by indicating that this is how "psychological and other diagrams become 'mandalas' and 'magic figures!'" (p. 46).

Chapter Seven

to functions of the circle or, more dynamically, to cyclical functions. Henry concludes that the most beautiful, most rhythmic figures are the circle or any of the polygons which can be derived from and inscribed within a circle. This includes the triangle, the square, or any of the more complex polygons whose angles are rhythmic with regard to the formula 2, 2^n, 2^n+1, or the sum of any of these numbers. These numbers, of course, are calculated in terms of the degrees of the circle. An excellent example of this formula is seen in the representation of the *chakras,* the psychic centers of the body which are traditionally symbolized by circles or circular forms with various geometrical figures derived from and inscribed within the circles.[12]

Essential to the circle is the center point, however that may be defined. Henry's biopsychic norm is simply represented by a circle and its center point. Writing in this tradition, Parmenides says that "being is like the mass of a well-rounded sphere whose force is constant from the center in any one direction."[13] For Borges, this metaphor recalls the famous statement, "God is an intelligent sphere whose center is everywhere and whose circumference is nowhere."[14] And Fechner declares that, as perfect beings, angels have a spherical form.[15]

12. See, for instance, Arthur Avalon, *The Serpent Power, Being the Sat-Cakra-Nirupana and Paduka Pancaka* (Madras, 1964; first edition, 1918), especially plates 1–8; see also Mookerjee, *Tantra Art.*

13. Jorge Luis Borges quotes this passage in his most suggestive essay, "Pascal's Sphere," in *Other Inquisitions,* p. 5.

14. Ibid., p. 6, attributed to Alain de Lille (Alanus de Insulis) who discovered it in the twelfth century in a text supposedly written by Hermes Trismegistus entitled *Asclepius.* As we have already suggested, Henry was himself an alchemist, a "hermetic" philosopher. For a contemporary text on the subject, I suggest that of M. Berthelet, a famous chemist, *Les Origines de l'alchimie* (Paris, 1885).

15. This is the idea developed in Fechner's "Anatomy of Angels," a supposedly comical book written under Fechner's satirical pseudonym of Dr. Mises (*Vergleichende Anatomie der Engel,* 1825). Yet in a "serious" work, *Ueber die Seelenfrage,* published in 1861, a year after the publication of the *Elements of Psychophysics,* Fechner writes: "It is true that solid

Signac's Portrait of Fénéon

Related to this general but pervasive idea is the concept of the mandala, which literally means "circle,"[16] and interestingly enough, in Tibetan translations, means either "center" or "that which surrounds."[17] Tucci describes the mandala as "map of the cosmos."[18] It is the symbol of psychophysical integration. This is naturally *similar* to the place of the circle/sphere in the Western hermetic tradition which Henry postulated in his conception of the biopsychic norm.

Furthermore, in the tradition of Henry's research, Metzner and Leary have recently indicated that the

> mechanism of the mandala can also be understood in terms of the neurophysiology of the eye . . . [indeed] the mandala is a depiction of the structure of the eye, the center of the mandala corresponds to the foeval "blind spot." Since this "blind spot" is the exit from the eye to the visual system of the brain, by going "out" through the center, you are going *in* to the brain. The Yogin finds the mandala in his own body. The mandala is an instrument for transcending the world of visually perceived phenomena by first centering them and then turning perception inward.[19]

---

and spherical angels are not to our liking, but to us this is incongruous only because we have been taught in the schoolroom to think of the earth as a papier-mâché globe." This suggests that the planet earth is itself one of the angels; the idea is really not so far away from the evolutionary view of the planet as a living organism developed by the late Teilhard de Chardin in the *Phenomenon of Man* (New York, 1959).

16. I paraphrase here the definition given by Mircea Eliade in *Yoga: Immortality and Freedom* (New York, 1958), p. 219. Another Western author who has written at length on the mandala is C. G. Jung, see particularly the publication Jung undertook with the sinologist Richard Wilhelm, *The Secret of the Golden Flower* (London, 1931). See also Jolande Jacobi, *The Psychology of C. G. Jung* (New Haven, 1942), pp. 131ff.

17. Eliade, *Yoga*.

18. Giuseppe Tucci, *The Theory and Practice of the Mandala* (London, 1961), p. 23.

19. Ralph Metzner and Timothy Leary, "On Programming Psychedelic Experiences," *Psychedelic Review*, no. 9 (1967):9. The relationship between the psychophysics practiced and formulated by Henry and that of psychedelics is quite clear, for the theory of dynamogeny is essentially no differ-

Chapter Seven

Certainly, one may consider Henry's *Cercle chromatique,* and its application in the *Portrait of Fénéon,* as the psychomathematical formulation of the transcendental yet omnipresent phenomenon of the mandala. This follows logically from Henry's idea that "from the point of view of consciousness, the form of the movements of expression is circular."[20] In Henry's phraseology it could be said that the mandala is a symbolic representation of the biopsychic norm: the unity of space, time, knowledge, and sensation—truly a "map of the cosmos."

This is something of what is contained in and suggested by the enamel ground "rhythmic with beats and angles, colors and tones" in the *Portrait of Fénéon:* a psychophysical vision of perceived form and of perception itself turned inward, as it were, revealing the vast kaleidoscope of ever-changing Mind.

---

ent than that of the expansion of consciousness. This is further suggested by Metzner himself in a review of C. Daly King's, *The States of Human Consciousness* (King was a Gurdjieff pupil), where Metzner states that King's book "stands in the tradition of Gustav Fechner and William James. It is an attempt to work out a systematic psychological theory of consciousness" (*Psychedelic Review,* no. 4 [1964]:486). It is to this tradition that Henry belongs with regard to modern psychological thought, the tradition of the psychology of consciousness.

20. See above, n. 7.

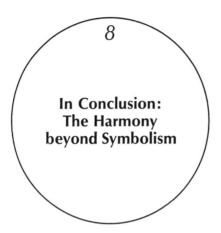

8

In Conclusion: The Harmony beyond Symbolism

PSYCHOPHYSICS, as Henry conceived and worked with it, is essentially a metaphor for harmony or the pursuit of harmony, whether this pursuit be defined as a science or an art. Harmony is a general condition which Henry was fond of evoking, and one might well consider him a harmonist: one, who in his own way, espouses the doctrine of harmony. As such, Henry is the heir to, and transmitter of, a seemingly ageless tradition, yet a tradition capable of ceaseless transformation. Psychophysics is thus a temporal manifestation of the doctrine of harmony.

In this light, Henry's role becomes much more clearly defined: that of articulating as best he could in the contemporary language, knowledge system, and formulas, the laws of harmony. Harmony is fundamentally an aesthetic idea, and for this reason any articulation of the laws of harmony finds its true realization in those works that are integral expressions of the laws of harmony and which are commonly called works of art. A corollary idea to the perennial philosophy of harmony is that of a perennial artistic tradition, whatever the technique used, expressive of harmony. Henry alludes to such an artistic tradition in speaking of contemporary symbolism in general: "Yes, I would be disposed to seeing in it [symbolism], perhaps more precisely put, the intuition of a new art. But the intuition of this art is of all times. It is in the *Vita Nuova* of Dante, and in the Spanish mystics, and in all the pages which are classically embedded in this point of view."[1]

In setting forth the doctrine of psychophysical aesthetics, Henry was merely calling attention to the psychophysiological premise of the *experience* of harmony, an experience known to the symbolists as "synesthesia." Moreover, although Henry expressed his basic ideas during the time of the symbolists in the 1880s and 1890s (the reason my study of the formation of a psychophysical aesthetic has been essentially devoted to this period), the applicability and influence of these ideas extends beyond the symbolist epoch well into the twentieth century. Indeed, one may posit a stream of art flowing from this time and directly related to the aesthetic doctrine of a psychophysical harmonics. Though this is no place for a detailed description and analysis of the harmonic stream of twentieth century art, or for the more general applications of the notion of psychophysical harmonics, I would like to indicate, however briefly, some aspects of the influence of the psychophysical aesthetic.

Let me first sum up the psychophysical aesthetic as articulated by Henry. Starting from the premise that what is real is sensation, sensation is then related to a general law of psychomotor reactions; these reactions can be reduced to the fundamental biopsychic principles of dynamogeny and inhibition and the corresponding mental functions of contrast, rhythm, and measure; these functions constitute the nature of consciousness; from the point of view of consciousness the form of the movements of expression is circular or, kinesthetically, cyclical. Finally, emphasizing the fundamentally psychophysiological character of this formulation of the aes-

1. "Enquête sur l'évolution littéraire," *L'art moderne* (October 25, 1891), p. 344.

The Harmony beyond Symbolism

thetics of harmony as it applies to the visual arts, Henry stated in 1922 that

> "it is possible to envision clearly and to anticipate within psychobiologcal functions light, color, and form. The properties of sensitive, motor, secretive, and trophic irritability are universally the same, excepting some secondary differences. This is why art, which is necessarily founded on the laws of our sensations, moves us so profoundly and gives us, moreover, so forcefully the illusion of life . . . the artist, if he has an exceptionally organized eye, feels and applies unconsciously the laws of normal sensitivity.[2]

Henry's aesthetic generally tends to be more far-reaching than could be acknowledged or realized by his contemporaries. The idea that art might be a regulated psychobiological projection of an unconscious nature, as is indicated in the last quote, is quite unique. Perhaps the most notable collective example of an art that is a more or less unconscious projection of psychobiological properties is art nouveau. Schmutzler refers to a "biological romanticism" as a quality of art nouveau form.[3] This can be taken quite literally as rhythms and biological visions felt and applied unconsciously, expressing life at its most fundamental level, yet not without its transcendental qualities as manifest in the general level of abstraction—undulating lines, rhythmically and dynamically manifested. Indeed, Schmutzler speaks of the "abstract dynamism" of art nouveau:

> Representational Art Nouveau had been attracted to the lower or primal organisms, but Van de Velde and abstract High Art Nouveau embody the dynamics of the elements of life itself, suggesting Henri Bergson's *élan vital,* that eternal energy which continues its uninter-

2. "La lumière, la couleur, et la forme," *L'Esprit nouveau* (1921), p. 1075.
3. *Art nouveau* (New York, 1964), pp. 260ff.

rupted pulsation, regardless of the stage of metamorphosis in which it happens to find itself, and of the particular form assumed by any species at any given time.[4]

As I have already indicated, however, Van de Velde was quite probably influenced by Henry's formulation of this eternal energy and its pulsations in the doctrine of dynamogeny and inhibition. Art, performing its proper life function, dynamogenizes; in this lies the very essence of the most predominant characteristic of art nouveau, the flowing line. As early as 1885, Henry spoke of the line as the abstraction of the reality of directions, and this idea is further developed in the *Cercle chromatique* to include the idea of curvilinear functions, so manifest in the *Portrait of Fénéon*.

Further examples of art as an unconscious projection of psychobiological functions and in which there is quite probably the influence of Henry are to be seen in the work of the Delaunays and Frank Kupka. Some clue of this influence is given by one writer who states that Henry "lent his arguments to the theories of the divisionists, and gave to diverse families of cubism certitudes supporting the most fantastic demonstrations."[5] Orphism and its impact is certainly one of these "families of cubism." This is evident in Delaunay's pronouncement, "On Light" (1913), which is much like a poetic echo of Henry's psychobiological ideas. Delaunay states that it is

> the simultaneity of light, the harmony, the rhythm of colors which creates the Vision of Man. Human vision is endowed with a greater Reality, since it comes to us from a direct contemplation of the Universe. The eye is the highest sense organ, that which communicates *con-*

4. Ibid., p. 272. It might be argued that Henry's formulation of the theory of dynamogeny and inhibition is merely a more precise statement of the *élan vital* of Bergson. In any case, the two concepts are not mutually exclusive.

5. René-Jean, "Hommage à Henry," pp. 54–55.

sciousness most directly to the brain. The idea of the vital movement of *the world and that movement itself are simultaneous.* Our understanding is correlative to our perception. *Let us seek to see.*[6]

In this respect, it is interesting how Delaunay's ideas, so obviously related to those of Henry, especially as expounded in the *Cercle chromatique,* also are reminiscent of an earlier harmonist, Plotinus, who remarked:

> It is first of all necessary to make the organ of vision analogous to the object to be contemplated. Never would the eye have perceived the sun if it had not first taken the form of the sun; likewise, the soul cannot see beauty unless it first becomes beautiful itself, and every man must make himself Beautiful and Divine in order to attain the sight of Beauty and Divinity.[7]

This is simply a mystical phrasing of the idea that the artist is he who with an exceptionally organized eye is able to project forth unconsciously, or intuitively, as it were, the inner psychobiological forms of beauty which are analogous to outer natural forms, as the circle is to the sun. As early as 1906, Delaunay turned to the circle/sun motif in a brilliant work which is one of that artist's first breaks away from the strict mosaic divisionism style exemplified by Signac at this time. This idea reaches its culmination in those works of the 1911–14 period emphasizing the circle, and the sun and moon. Aniela Jaffe relates one of the Delaunay sun and moon paintings of this time to the mandala motif in twentieth-century art as an expression of the impulse to wholeness or in-

6. Robert Delaunay, "La lumière," in *Du cubisme à l'art abstrait,* ed. Pierre Francastel (Paris, 1957), p. 146. "La lumière," written in 1912, was translated by Paul Klee into German and published in *Der Sturm* (1913), pp. 144–45.

7. From the *Enneads,* quoted in Jean Arp, *On My Way* (New York, 1948), p. 51.

tegrity.[8] The idea of wholeness or harmony is beautifully summed up by Henry: "The conscious concordance of an exterior mode of action and of a mode of representation constitutes the truth."[9]

In this vein, Kupka wrote in 1921:

> When the objective of painting becomes the exteriorization of intimate psychic events sustained only by such-and-such a source impression, this latter aspect figures in the painting only as a subject; however fixed it may be in reality, it no longer plays any role in painting. And this subject, whose true aspect has thereby lost its identity, no longer has any reason to be.[10]

Herein lies a formulation of abstract art that expresses the idea of psychobiological projection even more strongly than Delaunay did, and that, again, is very much in line with Henry's thought. Evidently, Henry's ideas and writings influenced Kupka most profoundly at the time the artist was evolving his first abstractions, entitled, significantly enough, the *Discs of Newton,* from 1908 to 1912. The works of Kupka which tend to be evocative of dynamic and even biological forms certainly exemplify the unconscious projection of psychobiological states. Indeed, abstraction in the art of Kupka and Delaunay can be viewed as an attempt at expressing the laws which govern the processes of consciousness and perception, much in the manner of Henry's mathematical abstraction of these laws into circles, cycles, and functions derived therefrom, with the intention of creating a more intense and yet expanded or dynamogenized sense of reality.

To further emphasize Henry's role in the formation of the first phase of twentieth-century abstract art, mention should

8. Aniela Jaffe, "Symbolism in the Visual Arts," in C. G. Jung, *Man and His Symbols* (New York, 1964), p. 247.

9. *Cercle chromatique,* p. 147.

10. Quoted in Paris *Kupka* (Paris: Musée de l'art moderne, 1966), p. 92.

be made of the group known as the *Section d'or,* which included the Duchamp brothers, Gleizes, Metzinger, Picabia,
and Léger, as well as the poet Apollinaire, and which was
frequented by Kupka.[11] The name of the group is itself most
suggestive of Henry, who stated in the *Cercle chromatique*
that the Golden Section was one of the basic dynamogenous
proportions. The name "Orphism," coined by Apollinaire, is
also suggestive of Henry's theory of dynamogeny, with its
overtones of musical, mystical ecstasy. This is also true of the
name and technique of the group known as the synchromists,
so obviously a reference to the theory of the simultaneous
contrast of colors, the most general principles of which were
so elaborately expounded in the *Cercle chromatique.* Of the
members of the Section d'or, Albert Gleizes apparently became most closely acquainted with Henry and in 1930 contributed an essay, "Charles Henry, universitaire," to the *Hommage à Henry.*[12] Finally, in outlining at least the extent of
Henry's influence in the first phase of twentieth-century abstraction, it is of significance that the translation of Delaunay's
"On Light" that appeared in *Der Sturm* in 1913 was by Paul
Klee.

From this brief review of Henry's influence on twentieth-
century art it should be evident that his theories contributed
significantly to the formation of the aesthetic base of what

11. See Chipp's article, "Orphism and Color Theory," pp. 55–63, which
discusses briefly Henry's influence on Delaunay, Kupka, and the Section
d'or.

12. Albert Gleizes, "Hommage à Henry," pp. 112–27, discusses at
length Henry's later research in terms of its revolutionary consequences for
the knowledge system of the West and with particular regard to the an-
tagonism that Henry's ideas and research created in the official university
community; no mention is made of the art events ca. 1908–14, though
Gleizes is obviously very partisan and acquainted with Henry's thought
and its metaphysical, anti-establishment orientation. Indication of Gleizes'
own artistic orientation is his pamphlet, *La mission créatrice de l'homme
dans le domaine plastique,* a reprint of a speech given to the Paris Theosophical Society, December, 1921.

has come to be called abstract art. On the other hand, acknowledgment of his influence on this development of modern art calls forth a reevaluation of the meaning and intention of the phenomenon of abstraction, if only because the role of psychophysics, which through Henry plays such an important part in the formation of modern aesthetic ideas, has in its entirety been quite neglected and overlooked.[13] Primarily, it is the art of the Delaunays, of Kupka, of the Section d'or, even of the futurist Severini, who was so influenced by the divisionism of Seurat, and to some extent of Paul Klee and Kandinsky, particularly after the twenties, that forms what I would call a base for a harmonic or dynamogenous stream of art in the twentieth century. Essentially this is a constructive, integrative artistic attitude based to a greater or lesser extent upon some knowledge of the perceptual functions of contrast, rhythm, and measure. In this sense, too, it can be said that there is a harmonic stream of art that extends beyond Henry's immediate influence since any art based upon knowledge of perceptual functions, with the end of creating a more harmonious, integrated state of consciousness, would be psychophysically harmonic. The work of Albers, much of "Op" art, and especially psychedelic art (in many ways so reminiscent of art nouveau) may be said to comprise the later stream of harmonic, psychophysical art. It should also be apparent that this kind or stream of art is not of the purist "art-for-art's sake" variety, but has a peculiar kind of utility, even if only by giving the eyes a retinal massage. Expressing the function of this kind of art, the psychophysiologist Jaensch wrote in 1922 that "art . . . is an attempt to revert from the disintegration induced by civilization to organic

13. Thus, for instance, Michel Seuphor, one of the leading firsthand authorities on the subject of earlier twentieth-century abstract painting, makes no mention of Charles Henry or psychophysical doctrines in his significant work, *L'art abstrait* (Paris, 1948). As far as I know, my account is the first to give some consideration to the significance of Henry's psychophysical ideas upon the formation of the first wave of twentieth-century abstraction.

modes of being."[14] Implicit in this, of course, is the idea of an art not restricted to any one style or technique.

Yet insofar as Henry was an exemplar of the harmonic mode, certain other aspects of his doctrine must be considered in order to determine ways in which his views or prophecies still have a validity today and may provide further clues to future developments in the art of harmony. Thus, in a statement from an interview which has been previously quoted and which bears repeating in view of the many interpretations surrounding "abstract art," Henry declared:

> I do not believe in the future of naturalism, or of any realistic school. On the contrary, I believe in the more or less imminent advent of a very idealistic and even mystic art based on new techniques. . . . I believe in the future of an art which would be the reverse of any ordinary logical or historical method, precisely because our intellects, exhausted by purely rational efforts, will feel the need to refresh themselves with entirely opposite states of mind.[15]

It should be evident that the various strands of abstraction extending from around 1910 through the 1920s, which I have indicated above, relate to some extent to Henry's idea of a very idealistic and even mystic art.

While Henry provides the seedbed for many of the perceptual formulations of the first wave of abstract art, the Theosophical doctrines of people like Madame Blavatsky and Rudolph Steiner seem to have given much of this art at least the patina of a mystical content.[16] Yet it is questionable to

---

14. In *Eidetic Images,* which is a fascinating study of an area of perception that is literally a borderline region where all possibilities are met: "Optical perceptual (or eidetic) images are phenomena that take up an intermediate position between sensations and images . . . they are ideas that, like after-images, are projected outward and literally seen" (pp. 108–9). It is still the best study of the phenomena.

15. "Enquête sur l'évolution littéraire," p. 343.

16. Peter Fingestein, "Spirituality, Mysticism and Non-Objective Art," *Art Journal* 21, no. 1 (Fall, 1961):1–6, broaches this thematic topic, though

Chapter Eight

what extent much twentieth-century abstract art satisfies the idea of an art that uses the reverse of logical or historical methods and is capable of refreshing intellects exhausted by purely rational efforts. Certainly, if nothing else, Henry put his finger on a present-day artistic/social dilemma. Insofar as society is rationally/technologically organized, with the deployment of large masses of people in automated, semi-automated, or purely cerebral labor, and insofar as the psychophysical ideal of art is that of providing and furthering a *harmonious* social arrangement through the creation of artistic vehicles for the release of energy in an *integrative* and constructive manner, then there is indeed much that has yet to be accomplished, or at least much that is wanting. Perhaps the difficulty lies in the fact that it is next to impossible for a society to create anything but a mirror of itself, at least given the present expectations and demands placed upon art and artists. Despite the advent of such new techniques as the cinema, such new materials as plastics, and such new environmental situations as light shows and rock concerts, more often than not one is not refreshed by an "opposite state of mind" but overwhelmed by a magnification or intensification of the existing state. What is lacking may be a widespread development of a new mode of consciousness, a mode not so much antithetical to the previous mode as one capable of synthesizing it and including it in its set of operations—a mode which would be to rational logic what rational logic is to instinct. Only then would there be possible the appearance of a mystic art which would be the reverse of any ordi-

---

obviously it could be treated with much greater thoroughness. Of the early abstractionists influenced by Theosophy, Fingestein mentions Kandinsky and Mondrian. It is clear that Kupka and Gleizes (see above, n. 14) were also intimately involved with this spiritual doctrine, and certainly we can surmise that its influence was rather pervasive in the first two or three decades of the twentieth century. Indeed, the Theosophical publication *Thought Forms* (1901) by Annie Besant and C. W. Leadbeater contains illustrations and ideas that formally are "abstract" and which precede by almost ten years the era of the great nonrepresentational breakthrough.

nary logical or historical method, capable of utilizing new techniques in a way appropriate to them and conducive to that dynamogenous state which Henry so emphatically professed, a state in which the individual's rhythm would harmonize with that of the collectivity to the same degree that the rhythm of the collectivity would harmonize with that of the individual.

To Henry it was evident that the social situation had to change in order for art to change in its technique as well as its content, though obviously the implementation of an art based upon psychophysical principles and emphasizing a harmonic and elevating sense of order and unity would be of the greatest benefit to the existing society. Some idea of this is given when Henry states:

> It is evident—is it not—that the dramas which consist in general of misunderstandings and mistaken identities will no longer make any sense in a given period of time: the fairy tale will replace, advantageously moreover, these psychological acrobatics. The love stories which we hear over and over again make sense only because of our social situation, which places a very small number of females in contact with a very small number of males, and which has need of circumscribing, with protective laws and particular guarantees, the act of love. It is obvious that all of this will become incomprehensible when society is organized otherwise.[17]

This comment, though more specifically concerned with literature, is interesting in its notion of fairy tales replacing the involved psychodramas of the day (which still prevail). Essentially there is even more to this idea, for the fairy tale, as is well known, is a story with a generally more profound psychological content than the modern romance. Furthermore, the fairy tale is capable of moving the consciousness of the organism more deeply precisely because of its enchanting

17. "Enquête sur l'évolution littéraire."

153

remoteness which, with its lack of any immediate threat, absorbs the organism the more intensely into it; thus one attains much more readily through the medium of the fairy tale (or myth) identification with the great archetypes or archetypal situations. Such identification, from Henry's point of view, is most dynamogenous because it reaches beyond the immediate personal self. What results is an expansion of awareness through the release of deep-seated energies which express themselves in a rhythmic sense of enlivenment. In this respect the myth or fairy tale is akin to harmonic art though not necessarily to abstract art, at least not insofar as abstract art remains a function of purely rational intentions. The most severely rational art will eschew all sense of evocation; but without the sense of evocation of realms beyond the rational, there is no dynamogenous quickening of the highest life-impulse, and in order for art to be of evolutionary service it must appeal to this sense of expanding awareness. A work like Walt Disney's *Fantasia* may yet be the most perfect, the most successful, and the most universal in its appeal of all the harmonic artistic efforts in the twentieth century. Certainly it is a perfect psychophysical vehicle, utilizing the technique of cinema in a truly flowing, cinematic way, creating startling combinations of synchronized visual/musical abstracts interwoven with fairy tales. This work may be considered close to the fulfillment of the symbolist *gesamkunstwerk* ideal. But *Fantasia* is an isolated flower. Finally a new mythology must arise, complementary to the new consciousness of which I have already spoken. From this, or rather interdependently developed with this, will arise that dynamogenous art which will totally give and inform, much as the cathedrals of the Gothic period. Who knows if this dynamogenous form will even be called art, but will be instead a super-mental environment? Some hint of this is apparent in Henry's own words:

I see in the future men fatigued by integral calculus, the problems of distribution and so forth, who will seek repose in physical and moral hydrotherapy; yes, due to the extraordinary contention, their brains will need for their repose baths of very cosmic, universal and elevated moral sentiment, idylls from which all reality and all contingencies will be banished.[18]

To succeed, such "baths" would have to have a multisensory appeal, indeed, a total sensory appeal, based upon an understanding of the psychophysiological functionings of the human organism. A total harmonic keyboard for the human body would have to be worked out based upon and utilizing the laws of contrast, rhythm, and measure. Some idea of this is suggested in Henry's *Essai de généralisation de la théorie de rayonnement:*

There are, equally, sensations complementary to one another. Electromagnetic sensations (colors, odors, and smells) and gravitational sensations are complementaries of the genital sensation which abolishes them when it is intense; reciprocally, the genital sensation is diminished when the former sensations are more intense (exception is made for smells of a sexual origin, musk, civet, etc.). The simultaneous excitation of the genital sensation and the electromagnetic sensations (especially visual and olfactory) provoke the equivalent of an excitation of the complete nervous field, analogous to the sensation of physiological white, provoked only by a pair of complementary colors, whereas the sensation of *physical* white requires the conjunction of all the visible colors; this pseudo-total excitation of the total nervous field would appear to define that which literature and current language understand by the word "love."[19] Internal sensations (hunger, thirst) are notoriously complementaries of the musical sensation. Recip-

18. Ibid.
19. Charles Andry-Bourgeois notes that Henry's last publication was actually entitled *Au-delà de l'amour (fréquences nerveuses des fonctions psychiques).* See Ch. Andry-Bourgeois, *L'oeuvre de Charles Henry et le problème de la survie* (Paris, 1931), p. 6.

rocally, the excitation of music and the appropriate locomotion, combined with that of a young perseverant, determines the nervous exaltation well known by the dervishes.

The functions which have complementaries are normally the reflexes of sensations perfectly determined: locomotion, sensation in general, more particularly, hearing, reproduction, genital sensation, assimilation (digestion), the electromagnetic and gravitational sensation, static work (active immobility), internal sensations (hunger, thirst); sleep has no persistent complementary.[20]

Because of this, Henry goes on to say, paraphrasing Wundt,

> . . . *only conscious are those sensations having complementaries*. As sensations are by definition characterized by consciousness, they imply a complex organization of elementary resonators reacting one upon the other successively and in an inverse way as well; *consciousness is a sensorial and psychic aspect of biological autoregulation*.[21]

Thus Henry envisioned that art would also function at least as an adjunct to therapy, whether physical or psychic, since the aim in any case is that of "bringing forth conscious processes where once there were but unconscious impulses and of restoring the organism to a state of harmonious autoregulation." As Henry comments, "There is fundamentally only one therapy."[22]

These concepts may be far from the conventional notions of art and may be looking far into the future. Yet the notion of art as a dynamogenous, integrating restorative, appealing to the totality of the organism's functioning and giving to the organism a sense of its own cosmic place, is one that has a function in a world that is still torn asunder by its own per-

20. *Théorie du rayonnement,* p. 196.
21. Ibid., p. 198.
22. Ibid.

sistent disharmonic functionings. Indeed, there can be seen here the base for a truly global vision or, rather, a vision of a truly global art in the sense that the psychophysical aesthetic deals fundamentally with the functions and properties of the human organism in its universality. Such an art would be a science as well, and its aim would be the restoration of that relationship or set of relationships by which man knows himself to be an integral, rhythmic, and interdependent aspect of the cosmos. Through such an art, man would be able to realize himself as *the* microcosm; and this is the age-old dream of harmony.

To those who would question the probability of arriving at such a vision, Henry provides the final appropriate comment:

> There are no fixed "canons" [of beauty]; there are an infinite number of them, all necessarily obedient to the laws of life. Within each race at each moment of time, each artistic temperament, chooses the rhythm of sensitivity appropriate to it. . . . This means that beauty is an evolutive phenomenon, that even the essential verities which constitute the principles of our theories are not learned—they are created.[23]

23. "La lumière, la couleur et la forme," p. 1075.

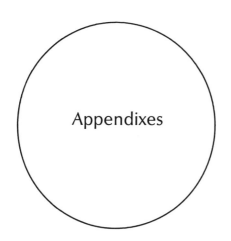

Appendixes

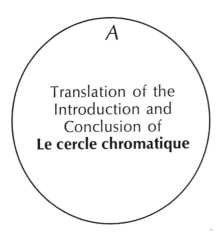

A

Translation of the
Introduction and
Conclusion of
Le cercle chromatique

Translator's note

The *Cercle chromatique* is probably Charles Henry's most significant general work both on psychophysics and aesthetics. Indeed, the psychophysical is inseparable from the aesthetic. In considering light, color, form, and sound, both as vibratory energy and as psychic functions, Henry inescapably formulates the basis of a psychophysical aesthetic. In the *Cercle chromatique*, Henry proved himself to be a moralist and a harmonist as well as a psychophysical aesthetician. In fact, the psychophysical aesthetic is the aesthetic of harmony in scientific dress. As Henry stated in the conclusion of the *Rapporteur esthétique* (published in conjunction with the *Cercle chromatique*), "to help the normal development of art is to favor as much the still distant realization of our destiny—the creation of universal harmony." It is to this end that Henry describes the various experiments and mathematical theories in the *Cercle chromatique*.

Henry believed that, given a general knowledge of the psychophysical nature and form of the sense elements, the artist could then construct works conducive to dynamogenous (as opposed to inhibitory) states of consciousness and ultimately to an amelioration of the social situation. Thus, in one of the later chapters of the *Cercle chromatique*, Henry

161

envisioned "the reality of a superior coordination of the virtual movements of individuals, just as the individual is a coordination of real movements of centers of an inferior order: the species then is quite really, and not metaphorically, an organism, but an organism of a virtual order, rhythmic or not, depending on whether the individuals are rhythmic or not . . . the development of the individual is then as impossible without the development of the species as the development of the species is impossible without the development of the individual." I can only hope that my translation of the often difficult passages of the Introduction and Conclusion of the *Cercle chromatique*—the first such translation into English—will give the reader some idea of the significance and flavor of Henry's thought.

J.A.

Introduction (extracts and résumés, preliminary ideas)

The observational and experimental method which, aided by calculus, has succeeded in astronomy and physics with brilliant and well-known results, is incapable of helping us know the molecular world, for the delicacy of these phenomena render experiments uncertain wherever they are possible. Providing facts, this method is a fortiori incapable of determining *that which ought to be,* that is to say, the normal character of living reactions.

I have succeeded in making precise that which can be understood as the *normal* and have founded on the necessary laws of our representations a method which offers to the fundamental hypotheses of the sciences all the certitude of which they are susceptible, and will permit us, without a doubt, to penetrate by these deductive processes into the infinitely minute molecular world. I have chosen the best studied excitations: lights, colors, forms, sounds. I have shown that the phenomena known under the name of *optical illusions, consonance, dissonance, modes,* and *harmony* are particular cases of subjective functions common to all ner-

Appendix A

vous reactions—*contrast, rhythm,* and *measure,* and I have seen that these functions permit the formulation of a law of organization, an ideal for living reactions. I have had manufactured instruments like the aesthetic protractor, and the chromatic circle which make possible the amelioration of forms and the harmonies of colors. Moreover the theory is general. Dynamogenous dumbbells, thermometers, and aesthetic pressure-gauges will soon, I hope, be applied in conjuring up the imminent dangers by which the abuse of destructive excitants and the ignorance of our true needs menace us. My method is essentially schematic, that is to say, adapted to the abstract and simplifying character of our representations.

That which is most important to psychic functions is continuity. When the thought flow ceases, there is fatigue; when the cessation is violent, there is suffering. We can define pleasure: the continuity of psychic functions; pain is the discontinuity of these functions. But we can only represent—and thus study scientifically—ourselves as movements: we must make precise what relation exists between psychic functions and movements.

Observation and reason show that the psychic functions can be considered as movements which have been or will be like virtual movements.

There is no sensation without an arrest of movement and, consequently, without a virtual movement in an inverse direction. If one focusses on an object without displacing the visual axis, and without closing the lids, the vision becomes indistinct. Reciprocally, a moderated movement of the luminous object makes vision much easier. If one touches an object without moving the finger, all notion of contact disappears after a few seconds. Vierordt[1] has demonstrated that

1. Hermann Vierordt (1853–1902), medical doctor and professor of physiology at Tubingen, published in 1881 *Das Sehen des Menschen* and in 1884 *Kurzer Abriss der Percussion und Auskultation,* long considered one of the standard texts on the subject (22d edition, 1930).

Appendix A

tactile sensitivity grows from the root of the member to its periphery, that it depends on the size of the movements, and that it is, for each segment of the member, proportional from the distance of the points of contact of the skin to the member's axis of rotation. There is no auditive sensation without a variation of the muscular tension of the tympanic membrane. If one sets in motion the tone la_3 to the extremity of a rubber tube hermetically fixed at the other end to the right ear, and if one attaches hermetically to the left ear a rubber tube transmitting the pressures of a Politzer insufflation bag, each light pressure effected on the bag to the left ear produces a light attenuation of the sound in the right ear; thus there is at the same time as the passive displacements the production of active movements, a synergetic action of accommodation in both ears. Thus, odor can only be experienced with the respiratory movements; taste, with the movements of the tongue.

Likewise, we can say that there is no idea without virtual movements becoming real movements. This is confirmed daily by the facts produced by instruments such as the plethismograph or Mosso's scales, which measure the modifications in the vascular phenomena in correlation with the slightest emotion. Thirty-four years ago, M. Chevreul rendered justice to the so-called exploratory pendules and divinatory rods in proving that observed movements—given the experiment of a ring suspended by a thread—are the products of unconscious muscular movements, the direction of which movements is determined by the corresponding idea.[2] The exactitude of these observations has been con-

2. The reference here is to the study by Michel-Eugene Chevreul (1786–1889), De la baguette divinitoire, du pendule dit explorateur et des tables tournantes (1854). A versatile scientist, Chevreul is known to art history as the publisher of De la loi du contraste simultané des couleurs et de l'assortiment d'objets colorés (Paris, 1839), though it is also interesting to note that in 1864 he published Des couleurs et de leurs applications aux arts industriels à l'aide de cercles chromatiques. In many ways, Henry's work is a further and more expanded realization of Chevreul's idea. See also

Appendix A

firmed. Recently, M. A. Charpentier drew attention to an optical illusion no less instructive.[3] When one regards for a period of time in complete darkness an immobile object of small diameter, dimly lighted, this object appears to move by itself. The angular speed of the apparent displacement is an average of 2° to 3° per second; the direction of the displacement is variable. Most often for the subject, the object appears to proceed along a curved line moving upward, and from within to without; these are the normal directions.[4] The total extension of displacement can attain and surpass 30°, that is, a twelfth of the circumference; these points should be

---

Faber Birren's recent reissue of the English version of Chevreul's work, *The Contrast and Harmony of Colors* (New Hyde Park, 1967).

3. Pierre-Marie-Augustin Charpentier (1852–1916), doctor, neuro-physiologist, published a variety of psychophysiological research studies, beginning in 1877 with a study of the emotional-sensorial excitations of the heart and including, in later years, a number of retinal-optical studies relating to light-sensitivity, photometry, the persistence of impressions, the speed of nervous reactions, and so on. Charpentier's research is typical psychophysiology for the period, and very closely related to Henry's work in this respect. As is evident from the experiments discussed by Henry, there is a great emphasis on the idea of the psychic nature of experience; what is of significance is that these experiments are presented as "evidence" supporting the law of psychomotor reactions: *"Every variation of physiological work is represented by real or virtual changes of direction of energy"* (*Cercle chromatique*, p. 14).

4. The idea of directions is crucial to an understanding of Henry's aesthetic. Direction, movement, change—psychophysically manifest as light, color, form, or sound—is the basic reality. Thus the first section following the Introduction to the *Cercle chromatique* deals with "interior work and directions" (pp. 11–24). The basic model of Henry's universe can be viewed as a continually self-transforming cycle or spiral, whose motivating mechanism is the ongoing exchange and transformation of energy from. one state to another, all states being complementary. Artistically applied, the theory of directions is the aesthetic-mathematical expression of the symbolist idea; psychically, the directions are transformed into symbols or, conversely, we only know directions symbolically. In this sense the directions are symbols, as it were, of sensory experience. Since for Henry the world *is* representation, it is primarily a symbol—or Baudelaire's "forest of symbols"—whose actual content is profoundly psychic in nature. The artist is he who realizes and actualizes the various symbols contained in the psyche.

Appendix A

well noted. It suffices to imagine seeing another object or to execute an act in another direction in order to provoke the apparent displacement of the object in this direction. The observer can voluntarily make his attention undergo small displacements in various directions around the object considered without ceasing to perceive the continuous movement of the latter in the original direction, and the illusion persists even in the indirect vision for all the points of fixation of attention. One can provoke the illusion of a determined direction while rubbing on the closed eye which does not partake of the experience. It is not the eye which accomplishes by itself the movement but, rather, the eye fixing its attention upwardly, the object would seem to proceed reciprocally downward. Let us suppose, on the contrary, simultaneous to the idea of a second object, for example, a closed door, the virtual taking into possession of this object by our organs of perception; then, the idea of the object changing, the organs will change place and the first object will be displaced in this direction.[5]

I could cite a great number of facts which denote, simultaneous with perception, the virtual realization of the object by our natural mechanics; but I believe it useless to insist on this point of view so familiar to contemporary psychology, so evident by itself, and without which it would be impossible, moreover, to understand anything of the suggestions of the idea brought about by the attitude and of the attitude by the idea.

In summing up, one can consider the sensation and the idea as virtual exercises of our natural mechanics: the sensation corresponds to a real movement which terminates in a virtual movement; the idea, to a virtual movement which is concluded in a real movement, but more or less quickly and

5. This entire idea is reminiscent of William Blake's concept:

If Perceptive Organs vary, Objects of Perception seem to vary:
If the Perceptive Organs close, their Objects seem to close also.
"Jerusalem"

under a different form, according to the nature of the subject.

The aesthetic problem is posed under a new form, and, this time, scientifically: "Which are the movements that the living being can describe continuously? Which are the movements that it can only describe discontinuously?" One sees that this problem does not depend on general mechanics, but on another mechanics which one could designate under the name of *situational mechanics*, the object of which has been made precise in this passage from a celebrated writing by Poinsot[6]: "Mechanics itself would present us with two kinds of mechanics; first, that which calculates the quantities of movements, the forces and speeds; then there is that which is seen only in the disposition of the bodies—their reciprocal play, the manner in which they develop their ways—and this without having avoided either the direction of these lines, or the time which the bodies take to describe them, or the forces which are necessary in order to move them."

On the other hand, this problem of the continuity and discontinuity of physiological movements is no different from the problem of dynamogeny and inhibition which has been posed in modern works, above all in the fine researches of M. Brown-Sequard.[7] According to the definition of this eminent physiologist, those nervous irritations are dynamogenous which, more or less instantaneously, for a duration more

6. Louis Poinsot, 1777–1859, geometrician, member of the French Academy of Sciences, author of the celebrated *Eléments de statique,* from which Henry takes the statement quoted in our text. Poinsot is considered one of the creators of static mechanics.

7. Charles Edward Brown-Sequard, 1817–94, eminent doctor and neurophysiologist, taught at Paris and Harvard; in 1878 succeeded Claude Bernard (under whom Henry studied in the middle 1870s) in the chair of experimental psychology at the College de France; in 1886 made president of the Biology Society of the Academy of Sciences. Brown-Sequard did a great deal of research on nervous and muscular systems and on the therapeutic methods pertaining to them; one of these therapies, opotherapy, is a pioneer form of organ transplant. It is to be noted that, in its application, Henry's aesthetic has a broadly therapeutic function: that of clearing up the sundry illusions to which the various sense organs are subject and which collectively create individual and social malaise.

Appendix A

or less long, in those nervous or contractile parts more or less distant from the place of irritation, will more or less exaggerate a function; those irritations are inhibitory which, under the same conditions, will more or less make a function disappear. The effects of inhibition are still known under the name of *phenomena of arrest*. The notion of discontinuity and the notion of arrest are identical: the notion of continuity is related to the idea of the acceleration of functions, and of accelerated movement being able to be considered as a movement whose continuity is augmented each instant. Everyone knows that to each agreeable sensation corresponds a growth in the available force, to each disagreeable sensation a diminution. These facts M. Feré[8] has made precise by measuring on a dynamometer, in hysterical patients as well as normal subjects, the variations of the force according to the nature of the sensation. Thus, with a certain Dr. G., the force of whose right hand varies from 50 to 55 kilograms, as soon as his nostrils are quickly approached by a flask of pure musk, he declares it disagreeable and sees his force lowered to 45 kilograms. If one places the flask at a certain distance, he declares the odor very agreeable, and the dynamometer registers 65. With a hysteric, the approach of the flask of musk determines a very agreeable sensation which is translated by a rise from 23 to 46 on the dynamometer.

One can thus consider as an absolute general range, aes-

8. Charles Feré, 1852–1907, contemporary psychophysiologist whose research Henry draws upon in the *Cercle chromatique*. In 1887, Feré published *Sensation et mouvement*. Related to the works of Henry and Feré on kinesthetics is that of Edouard Marey, 1830–1904, the developer of chronophotography—a predecessor of cinema, the art of film—friend of Henry and author of the *Étude de la locomotion animale par la chronophotographie* (Paris, 1887). The importance of the psychophysiological study of motion at this time cannot be stressed enough in its impact on altering the perception of nature from static to fluid and dynamic; this is particularly crucial for an understanding of the art of the 1890s—art nouveau—as well as the art of the first decades of the twentieth century. From impressionism to cubism, one witnesses a gradual disintegration of the classic one-point perspective system developed in the Renaissance.

Appendix A

thetic as well as physiological, the following problems: "Which are the movements the living being can describe continuously? Which are the forms that these conditions impose upon perception?"

Conclusion and Vocabulary

I have given all the developments necessary to a theory of visual sensation and to the illustration of a chromatic circle; as these particular problems could not be resolved without the general problem, I have been obliged to take up the aesthetic problem, so that I could get back to the scientific problem by this consideration, already evident to me under diverse forms; for the psychic functions are virtual movements, either continuous or discontinuous. I have studied the conditions of continuity and discontinuity, which are nothing other than the conditions of dynamogeny and inhibition of physiological functions, and I have mathematically made precise the forms of perception imposed by these conditions. The essential result is that our representations are necessarily cyclical in form, either continuous or discontinuous. As dynamogeny is only an emission of electricity, and inhibition an emission of heat or a raising of temperature, I have been able to make precise the intimate and evident liaisons within the living being in psychic phenomena such as pleasure and pain; in mechanical phenomena such as continuity and arrest; and in physical phenomena such as electricity and heat.

Furthermore, these modes of action are veritably irreducible[9] since they correspond to modes of irreducible and elementary representation. The study of the mechanism of potentials is thus an illusory problem. Accordingly, in the future there will be a greater precision, to the point at which cosmogonies and in general the so-called problems of origin

9. For Henry, unlike the physiologist Hermann von Helmholtz, the ultimate element of perception, be it for the organ of sight or sound, is irreducible and cannot be "explained." See Henry's article, "L'oeuvre ophthalmologique de Thomas Young," *La Revue blanche* 8 (1895):473–77.

will be something other than speculations as illegitimate as they are unjustifiable.

The last two chapters[10] are examples of this method of necessary representations, which, it seems to me, ought to be substituted for the speculations on energy and matter, for those inextricable hypotheses on ether and other subtle media, for the intuitions more or less falsified by the individual sickness and social milieux which constitute philosophy and the sciences. It is to these double reactions—continuity and discontinuity—that all scientific facts must finally be related, be they the subjective determinations which constitute mathematics, or the objective determinations which are the aim of the natural sciences. The first point of view has been presented by H. Wronski[11] and demands important developments in the general theory of functions; the second is pre-

10. The two chapters to which Henry refers deal with the nature of absolute thermal and electric measurements deduced from subjective functions, and the general equation of mechanics, which reads: "It is necessary and sufficient for the equilibrium and for all the possible systems of virtual movements, that the sum of reversible virtual movements be zero, and the sum of nonreversible virtual movements be zero and negative" (*Cercle chromatique*, p. 161).

11. Joseph-Marie Hoene-Wronski, 1778–1853, Polish mathematician philosopher, with whom Henry felt a great affinity (see Gustave Kahn, "Charles Henry: quelques souvenirs de jeunesse," *Cahiers de l'étoile*, no. 13 [January–February, 1930]:58). Having served with Kosciuszko and Dumbroski in the Napoleonic wars, Wronski had a revelation of the "higher truth" in 1803 and resolved to dedicate the rest of his life to the dissemination of that higher truth of which he felt himself the repository. His publications include *Philosophie critique découvert par Kant* (1803); *Introduction à la philosophie mathématique* (1811); *Philosophie de l'infini* (1814); *Union finale de la philosophie et de la religion, constituant la philosophie absolue* (1831–39). Having emigrated to France, Wronski became a colorful character in his own right, appearing in Balzac's "Recherché de l'absolu" (*Martyrs ignorés*) as Grodninski, the philosopher who sells the absolute to a Parisian banker (taken from real life!). In any case, we must attribute Henry's synthesizing cosmic outlook to Wronski. Though Wronski's mathematical ideas appear in Henry's work, the only publication by Henry dealing specifically with the Polish mathematician is *Wronski et l'esthétique musicale* (Paris, 1887).

Appendix A

sented in the works of Maxwell,[12] Lorentz,[13] Wilhelm Weber,[14] and Kohlrausch,[15] who, by absolutely different ways, are agreed in demonstrating the presence of electric currents in luminous undulations, and in reducing all physical forces to electricity, to heat, and to universal gravitation.[16] As the representations of the living being are now related to these mathematical operations, it is possible to found on this subjective point of view a method of direct transformation of the expression of the facts into quantitative formulas. It is evident for all scholars worthy of the name that certitude in the sciences can be obtained only by a principle superior to the experiment: the inductive method, precious instrument of research in the extreme specialities, is only an instrument of truth on the condition of yielding finally to the deductive method. When Wronski thought of deducing from the abso-

12. Clerk Maxwell, 1831–79, important English physicist, the first to develop the idea of the electromagnetic nature of light and heat, confirmed by the experiments of Hertz. Henry was in the vanguard of thinkers in realizing the applications and implications of the then budding theories of radiation and quantum mechanics.

13. Hendrick Antoon Lorentz, 1853–1928, Dutch physicist who developed in the 1890s the electronic theory of matter and received the Nobel prize for physics in 1902.

14. Wilhelm Weber, 1804–91, professor of physics at Halle, Göttingen, Leipzig; with the mathematical physicist C. F. Gauss, 1777–1855, worked on the concept of terrestrial magnetism and invented a scientific system of magnetic and electric units based on the fundamental units of length, mass, and time.

15. Probably Rudolf Kohlrausch, 1809–58, German physicist at Göttingen, who published with Weber in 1857 *Electrodynamischen Massbestimmungen,* and who is the inventor of an early electrometer. Kohlrausch had a son, Frederick, 1840–1910, who also engaged in electrical research and published in 1888 *Ueber den absoluten elektrischen Leitungwiderstand des Quicksilbers.*

16. Here lies the seed of Henry's later lifework which culminated in the 1924 publication, *Essai de généralisation de la théorie de rayonnement: résonateurs gravitiques, résonateurs biologiques . . .* , in which he puts forth his universal field theory of ultimate interchangeability of the phenomena of nature whether biopsychic, gravitational, or electromagnetic; that is, all phenomena are variables of a universal quantum wave.

Appendix A

lute all human knowledge, past and to come, he was deceived, for the idea of the absolute is only a phenomenon whose affirmation and negation are subject to the laws of our organization.[17] His attempt could rest only on an intuition more or less complete of the law of our organization, and it would be within this law that the absolute would have to be sought, if an indefinitely evolutive law could be said to be absolute. Pythagoras felt it to be so; but his great intuition degenerated rapidly in speculations without issue. When Descartes founded on thought the principle of all certitude and related form to number; when Leibnitz completed the mathematical work of Descartes by a practical conception of infinity and strove to found a living and ordered dynamism; when Kant demonstrated space and time to be forms of perception, these great thinkers were obedient to the practice of notable simplifications and to that point of view which promises to the principles of science all the certitude of which they are susceptible.

Vocabulary

Continuity, discontinuity—property of an ideal movement of power, or lack of it, to be described without interruption in time and space: a cycle whose ideal radius symbolizes the radius of the circle-unity normally realized by the upper right or left appendages and is continuous; it is relatively discontinuous when its ideal radius symbolizes the radius of a maximum pseudo-cycle realized by the coordination of the upper and lower, right and left appendages; it is absolutely discontinuous when it is larger or smaller than any defined cycle, and that can be realized only by points or by instants in an ideal translation, more or less complete, of the center.

17. Here Henry probably refers to his general law of psychomotor reactions: the reduction of phenomena to that of psychophysical energy exchanges. See Henry, *Sur une loi générale des réactions psycho-motrice* (Paris, 1890), as presented at the Congrès de Paris de l'Association française pour l'avancement des sciences.

Appendix A

Contrast—subjective function which reduces the representations to certain types such as the complementary, and the relations to natural units, the groups of certain aggregates.

Evolution (law of)—law after which the successive representations tend to become simultaneous and reciprocal; a law which must not be forgotten at any point within this writing. One can construct the curve of evolution in the direction of time according to my fundamental theorem: purely successive groups being able to be represented by primary numbers, the successive groups becoming more and more complex will be symbolized by the sums of successive primary numbers. According to this law, each time that one of the sums will be able to be placed under the form of a product, it will tend to be realized under that form. Let us take on the x- and y-axis in equal lengths the series of numbers; let us make on the x-axis the sums of the primary numbers: $1+2=3$; $3+3=6$; $6+5=11$; $11+7=18$ . . . One sees that for the second and fourth successions [6 and 18] the sums are composed numbers: let us raise the perpendiculars in each of the points which correspond to the sum-products and to the product-sums, and let us join the different points of intersection; one then has the curve of the influence of time that I have related in my work to the curve of probable distribution of errors according to their order of size.

Functions of one side; two-sided functions—representations which are marked to the left *or* to the right; to the right *and* to the left, according to the degree of continuity or discontinuity and which consequently participate in the more or less precise laws to which analogous representations are subject.

Matter—after the principles already admitted, it is *that which is directed* in our representations, that is to say, the radii of an ideal cycle which can always be assimilated at some point of arrest, given that the cycle is only an ideal. The representa-

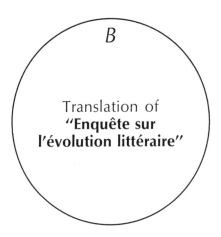

B

Translation of
**"Enquête sur
l'évolution littéraire"**

Translator's note
The depth of Henry's vision far exceeded common literary and artistic expectations: Some idea of this is evident in the following interview which appeared in 1891. Even today our arts but dimly aspire to the unitive vision glimpsed by Henry; and with the exception of the technical innovation of light shows and rock concerts, we are yet far from an art form which offers the transfiguring release of a physical and moral hydrotherapy. No doubt the future still belongs to M. Charles Henry.

With regard to the text itself, the "Inquiry Concerning the Future of Literature," was one of a series of interviews originated by the journalist, Jules Huret, and first appeared in *L'echo de Paris,* June, 1891; it was then reprinted in *L'art moderne* (October 25, 1891), pp. 343–44. My translation is taken from the latter text. The title in French is "Enquête sur l'évolution littéraire." Rewald, who prints part of this interview in *Post-Impressionism* (1956), p. 483, lists this as "Réponse à l'enquête de Jules Huret sur l'évolution de la littérature francaise." Rewald's translation is only of the first two paragraphs of Henry's response, and I therefore have the honor of reproducing in full the unusual vision contained therein.   J.A.

Appendix B

The Interview

M. Charles Henry is most notably the author of a scientific aesthetic which attempts to relate to our physiological organism the conditions and the laws of beauty. He is considered to have influenced in literature the most extreme and the most conscious of the symbolist decadents, such as Jules Laforgue[1] and Gustave Kahn;[2] and, in painting, the impressionists of the divided tone, notably Seurat and Signac.[3]

Mathematician and scholar, he has been able to put many of his discoveries into practice. This has merited him the approval of the scholarly world, the Academy of Sciences among others; his discoveries have also found their realization in various industrial projects. All of this has been inspired by a general scientific method, which has not yet been entirely formulated, and which has had the value of retaining the attention even of its adversaries.[4]

---

1. Jules Laforgue, 1860–87, perhaps one of the most significant of the symbolist poets, was also an outstanding art critic and a very close friend of Henry's, whose influence is most evident in Laforgue's essay on "Impressionism," first published in 1883, and recently republished in Linda Nochlin, *Impressionism and Post-Impressionism, 1874–1904* (New York, 1966), pp. 14–20. See above, chapter 4.

2. Gustave Kahn, 1859–1936, another close friend of Henry's; poet, critic and founder of the leading journals *La vogue* and *Les symbolistes,* his book of poetry *Les palais nomades* (1887) is reputed to be the first example of free verse.

3. Georges Seurat, 1859–91, and Paul Signac, 1863–1935, were most intimate with Henry in the 1880s, and their technique of the divided tone, "neo-impressionism" as it was dubbed by the critic Félix Fénéon, most certainly owes the accuracy of its technical finesse to the guiding influence of Charles Henry. This is most singularly borne out in the famous *Portrait of Fénéon* (1891) by Signac, though it is also most curious that in Signac's account of neo-impressionism (*De Delacroix au néo-impressionnisme* [1899]), there is not one mention of Henry—probably because at that time the latter had gone so far afield that Signac had difficulty in understanding all of the implications of Henry's theories. See above, chapter 7.

4. What Huret alludes to here is Henry's formulation of psychophysics; originated by the German philosopher/scientist Gustav Fechner in his 1860 publication *The Elements of Psychophysics,* this may be said to be the study of the transformation of external phenomena into states of consciousness and vice versa, though in actuality psychophysics today is ba-

Appendix B

Thirty years old, tall, thin, and loosely built, he physically fulfills the type of being called *ultra modern,* that type having in it all the effects of the long intellectual culture of the race. To see his streamlined hands, delicate, capable of subtle tasks, one easily imagines that the nervous fluid which makes them move in such an extraordinary fashion is of the most refined essence mortally possible. His general demeanor expresses the confidence of the scholar in the unlimited power of machines . . . he disdains having muscles. . . .[5]

In sum, he appears very rationally as the historiographer of our most refined sensations, which he weighs and measures and in which he discovers new worlds—a Des Esseintes both reasonable and wise.[6]

I asked him:
In which way do you think the future of literature will develop?

CH—I do not believe in the future of psychologism or naturalism, or in general of the whole school of realism. I believe, on the contrary, in the more or less imminent advent of a very idealistic and even mystical art, founded on absolutely new techniques. I believe this because we are witnessing a greater and greater diffusion and development of scientific methods and industrial efforts; the economic future of the various nations is involved in this, and social questions force us to follow this lead, for, after all, the problem of the pro-

sically the measurement of sense impressions. For Fechner as well as Henry, however, psychophysics, as the very name implies, was the basis for a system unifying mind and matter. See above, chapter 2.

5. Amusingly enough, the seemingly dapper Henry was an avid bicyclist, who wrote an amazingly involved series of articles for the *Revue blanche* in the 1890s on the psychophysiological aesthetics of bicycling; his most outstanding feat, however, was bicycling from Paris to Brussels and back.

6. Des Esseintes is, of course, the chief character in the novel *À rebours* (Against the grain) by Joris-Karl Huysmans, 1848–1907. This book, with its protagonist of ultimate esoteric and aesthetic delectation, was most aptly characterized by Arthur Symons as "the breviary of decadence."

Appendix B

gressive life of all people can be summed up thus: *produce much, cheaply, and in a very short time.*

Europe is obliged not to let herself be outrun or even annihilated by America, which has for a very long time combined its national education and its entire organization for the purpose of reaching this goal. I believe in the future of an art which would be the reverse of any ordinary logical or historical method, precisely because our intellects, exhausted by purely rational efforts, will feel the need to refresh themselves with entirely opposite states of mind. You need only look at the singular vogue of occult, spiritualist and other doctrines, which are misleading, because they can satisfy neither reason nor the imagination.

JH—Symbolism would appear to you as one of the manifestations of this new tendency?

CH—Yes, or perhaps more precisely, I would be disposed to see in it an intuition of a new art.

But the intuition of this art is of all times. It is in the *Vita Nuova* of Dante, and in the Spanish mystics, and in all the pages which are classically embedded in this point of view.[7]

Among the actual symbolists, several have understood, more or less vaguely, that outside of the logical boundaries of ideas there could be associative images inseparably founded on purely subjective laws. This is borne out in the fact that there can be intimate relationships between the hearing of certain sounds, the vision of certain colors, and the feeling of certain states of soul, inexplicable by objective concordances, and the basis of which is in the analogous echoes which these sounds, colors, and states of soul awaken in our organism.

To be more precise: there are relations between the vision of the direction going from below to above and the vision of the color red; between the vision of the direction from left

7. This idea of an "art of all times" was most beautifully pursued by Aldous Huxley in *The Perennial Philosophy* (New York, 1962).

178

Appendix B

to right and the color yellow. A red surface will appear higher, a yellow surface will appear wider, even though they may be of equal size.[8] For a long time now we have associated height with sharp sounds, and depth with low sounds—wrongly, moreover, for there is an index of reversal showing in the modern age a rather sensitive evolution in the tendency of the pitch towards sharp sounds.[9]

JH—Is there not an analogy between your theories and those of René Ghil?[10]

CH—The literary processes of M. Ghil certainly have no relation, neither close nor distant, with those of science. They are individual fantasies, constructed logically, which have any number of reasons for being incomprehensible. On the other hand, look at Rimbaud: right alongside a gigantic madness, intuitions of genius which go to the heart of all cultivated beings; his is a somewhat imprecise literary technique which presupposes the accomplishment of a psychophysiological refinement from which we are yet some distance. There will always be, furthermore, in the constitution of such a technique, difficulties stemming from the hereditary influence and special history of the individual which will determine perturbations frustrating to every kind of law.

From this follows, fundamentally, with such a technique,

8. Ideas of this nature are most exhaustively pursued in Henry's aesthetic magnum opus, the *Cercle chromatique* (1889).

9. This thought, rather obscurely expressed, was more fully developed by Henry in an article entitled, "Loi d'évolution de la sensation musicale," *La revue philosophique* (1886), pp. 81–87.

10. René Ghil, 1862–1925, poet and disciple of Mallarmé, wrote in 1886 the *Traité du verbe*, which, taking off from Rimbaud's famous poem, "Voyelles" ("Vowels"), develops an astoundingly intricate and mostly unscientific theory of "instrumentation," relating language to other sensations—colors, smells, and so on. On the basis of this, Ghil went on to write an elaborately complex epic, which is little remembered today. In his criticism of Ghil and in his praise of Rimbaud, Henry manages to put his finger on the fundamentally personal and emotional nature of the art of modern industrial societies, characteristics which seriously limit the scope of art.

a truly emotional art which of necessity will be an art more or less personal, more or less of the *cenacle* or group, and accessible only to beings who live the same moral life. This is the result, moreover, to which we have been led by all the necessities and social transformations of modern civilization. In effect, the more we progress the more we tend to uniformity. Look at England: everybody wears the same high hat, the coachman is a gentleman indistinguishable from the rest of his clients, save perhaps for something in his bearing; the same goes for the vendors of bread!

The progress of social organization will have the effect of simplifying and ameliorating our individual psychology. It is evident—is it not?—that the dramas which consist in general of misunderstandings and mistaken identities will no longer make any sense in a given period of time: the fairy tale will replace, advantageously, these psychological acrobatics. The love stories which we hear over and over again make sense only because of our social state, which places a very small number of females in contact with a very small number of males, and which has need of circumscribing the protection and particular guarantees of the act of love. It is obvious that all of this will become incomprehensible when society will be organized otherwise, with the children in the care of the state, for example. That is to say, woman will take herself integrally into her own possession, and, becoming free to choose, she will love the kind and number of men which are pleasing to her.

Then, as you will see, the necessary march of industrial and economic progress will lead us to a simplification in all things. . . .

JH—But language?

CH—Language likewise will be submitted to this evolution. Already there are striking examples; it is certain that we shall arrive at a stable state of language which will tend to a certain immobility in the evolution of psychological factors. I consider the evolution of language as due to the contradiction which is produced between the natural sounds of vowels and the tones of the voice which express the sentiment suggested by the word. . . .

JH—I don't quite understand.

CH—For example: the suggestion of an exciting sensation by an idea the word for which is composed of bass vowels such as *u* or *ou* will inevitably determine the transformation of the vocable in the higher vowels; it is thus that the transformation from *pater* to *père* has been able to be made. *A* is a b flat of the third octave, *e* a b natural of the fourth, according to Helmholtz.[11] The idea which one used to have of paternity, has it not evolved? But it would take much too long to attempt to solve here a problem as complicated as this. In order to arrive at some precise notions in this area, I am working at this time on an apparatus for analyzing the modifications of the sounds emitted following the expression of a sentiment. I shall show it to you one of these days.

JH—Summing up then, how does the literature of the future appear to you?

CH—I see in the future men fatigued by integral calculus, the problems of distribution, and so forth, who will seek repose in physical and moral hydrotherapy; yes, the extraordinary turmoil of these brains will need for their repose baths of very cosmic, universal, and elevated moral sentiments, idylls from which all reality and all contingencies will be banished. . . .

11. H. L. F. von Helmholtz, 1821–94, famous nineteenth-century scientist, author of the standard *Handbuch der Physiologischen Optik* (1855–65) and a work on the sensations of tone, to which Henry undoubtedly refers here. For all of Henry's elaborate analysis of language, his final summation of the future of literature is most ironic, indeed.

Bibliography

The most important biographical source for the life and work of Charles Henry is the curious publication "Hommage à Henry," *Cahiers de l'étoile,* no. 13 (January–February, 1930), which includes twenty-two articles dedicated to Henry; among the contributors are Gustave Kahn, Paul Valéry, Paul Signac, and Albert Gleizes. Many of the contributions deal with Henry's life after the period which we are investigating, but shed much light on the character and nature of Henry's life-long endeavor: the creation of a theory which synthesizes all human knowledge and experience. The *Cahiers de l'étoile* was itself a journal dedicated to the reunion of mysticism and science, and the issue devoted to Henry sums up the editorial position of this journal. "We render hommage to Henry, conqueror of the Unity," the editors conclude in their introduction, which is followed by a poem by Krishnamurti, "Await Me, O Friend." Indeed, the picture of Henry which emerges from this "hommage" is fantastic: was Henry an incredible madman? And if he wasn't, if there is even a grain of truth in his work, and we have no reason to doubt this much, then certain of Henry's theories and discoveries are of a most far-reaching nature. For instance, one of his last projects was to catalyze the hydrogen atom in such a way that tremendous amounts of energy would be released. It was his aim to find the proper institution to handle his discovery and research, for he was well aware that, although he intended the release of energy from the hydrogen atom as a way of aiding humanity, such a potent energy source could just as easily be misapplied. It is also obvious now that Henry, in this case, was one of the pioneers of atomic energy and that the hydrogen bomb was exactly what he most feared if his research fell into the wrong

Bibliography

hands. As it is, what happened to Henry's work after his death is not clearly known. The day of Henry's death appears to have been November 3, 1926, in Versailles. The last part of Henry's life demands proper research.

In addition to the *Cahiers de l'étoile,* several books based largely on Henry's later work should be cited: Robert Mirabaud, *Charles Henry et l'idéalisme scientifique* (Paris, 1926); C. Andry-Bourgeois, *L'oeuvre de Charles Henry et le problème de la survie* (Paris, 1931); F. Warrain, *L'Oeuvre psychobiophysique de Charles Henry* (Paris, .1931).

More recently there is the article by J.-F. Revel, "Charles Henry et la science des arts," *L'Oeil,* no. 119 (November, 1964):20–27, 44, 56, which, although drawing together already published information concerning Henry in the 1880s and 1890s, really adds nothing new to the knowledge of Henry. Revel does publish a photograph of Henry, the only one I know of, but this is of Henry in his fifties.

In the special issue of *Les Cahiers de l'étoile* devoted to Henry, Paul Signac wrote, "The best homage that we can render him [Henry] is to publish without adjectives or superlatives the complete list of his publications and the enumeration of his scientific works." We attempt to do simply that, listing chronologically the publications of Henry; we do not pretend to completeness, though for the period up to 1895 we have tried to be as thorough as possible. J. F. Revel, in *L'Oeil,* has suggested that Henry's work can be put into four categories:

1. Scholarly and historical works.
2. Aesthetic writings.
3. Psychophysics—"mathematics of life."
4. Final synthesizing works—"psychobiophysics."

Revel's categories are helpful, though we have not attempted to utilize them in our list; furthermore, there is in our list a rough chronological correspondence to the categories of Revel, which is also of interest. In the future we should like to see published a full, annotated bibliography of Charles Henry, the master bibliographer. This of course would depend upon access to the papers, library, laboratory, and sundry documents of Henry, which we have not had.

1878   "Sur l'origine de la convention dite de Descartes." *Revue archéologique* 35 (1878):251–59.
        "Sur une première rédaction du *Traité de la connaissance*

Bibliography

de Dieu et de soi-meme de Bossuet." *Archives de Herrig.* Brunswick, 1878.

1879   "Sur l'origine de quelques notations mathématiques." *Revue archéologique* 37 (1878):324–33; 38 (1879):1–10.

Opusculum de Multiplicatione et Divisione Sexagesimalibus Diophanto vel Pappo Attribuendum Primo. Hallis Saxoniae: H. W. Schmitt.

"Sur une valeur approchée de $\sqrt{2}$ et sur deux approximations de $\sqrt{3}$." *Bulletin des sciences mathématiques.* Paris, 1879.

Un érudit homme du monde, homme d'église, homme de cour: Lettres inédites de Madame de Lafayette, de Flechier, de Bossuet, etc. à Huet. Paris, 1879.

Huygens et Roberval, documents nouveaux. Leyden, 1879.

1880   *Recherches sur les manuscrits de Fermat.* Rome, 1879–80.

"Sur divers points de la théorie des nombres." *Bulletin de l'Association française pour l'avancement des sciences.* Paris, 1880.

Mémoires inédites de ch.-Nic. Cochin sur le comte de Caylus, Bouchardon, les Slodtz. Paris, 1880.

Galilée, Torricelli, Cavalieri, Castelli: documents nouveaux. Rome, 1880.

1881   "Sur un procédé de division rapide." *Nouvelles annales de mathématiques.* Paris, 1881.

Étude sur le triangle harmonique. Paris, 1881.

1882   *Supplément à la bibliographie de Gergonne.* Rome, 1882.

Notice sur un manuscrit inédit de Mydorge. Rome, 1882.

Mémoires de calcul integral de Joachim Gomes de Souza. Publiées avec additions et notices. Leipzig, 1882.

Les deux plus anciens traités français d'algorisme et de géométrie. Publiés pour la première fois. Rome-Paris, 1882.

1883   *Correspondance inédite de Condorcet et de Turgot.* Publiée avec notices. Paris, 1883.

Les connaissances mathématiques de Jacques Casanova de Seingalt. Rome, 1883.

Problèmes de géométrie pratique de Mydorge. Enoncés et solutions publiés avec commentaires orientaux de M. Leon Rodet. Rome, 1883.

1884   *Sur les methodes d'approximation pour les équations differentielles.* Mémoire inédite de Condorcet, publiée avec une notice sur ses écrits mathématiques. Rome-Paris, 1884.

Bibliography

L'encaustique et les autres procédés de peinture chez les anciens. (With Henry Cros.) Paris, 1884.

1885   "Les manuscrits de Leonardo da Vinci: Manuscrits A et B de l'Institut," *Revue de l'Enseignement secondaire et superiéure.* January, 1885.

Pierre de Carcavy. Rome-Paris, 1885.

"Les microbes de l'atmosphère." *La revue contemporaine* 2 (1885):105–17.

Introduction à une esthétique scientifique. Paris: Librairie Hermann, 1885. Originally published in *La revue contemporaine* 2 (August, 1885):441–69.

1886   "Vision," published in first issue of *La vogue.* April, 1886.

"Théorie des directions." John Rewald, *Le Post-Impressionnisme* (Paris, 1962), p. 64, refers to such a work, as does Lövgren, *Genesis of Modernism* (Uppsala, 1959), p. 40, though we have been unable to confirm it.

Correspondance inédite de d'Alembert avec Cramer, Lesage, Clairaut, Turgot, Castillon, Beguelin, etc. Précédées d'une notice sur ses travaux mathématiques. Rome-Paris, 1886.

Lettres inédites de Mademoiselle de Lespinasse. Avec une étude et des documents nouveaux. Paris, 1886.

"Loi d'évolution de la sensation musicale." *La Revue philosophique* (1886), pp. 81–87.

1887   *Oeuvres et correspondances inédites de d'Alembert.* Publiées avec introduction, notes et appendice. Paris, 1887.

La théorie de Rameau sur la musique. Paris: Editions de La vogue, 1887.

Wronski et l'esthétique musicale. Paris: Publication de La vogue, 1887.

Voltaire et le Cardinal Quirini. Paris, 1887.

Introduction a la chymie. Manuscrit inédit de Denis Diderot. Publiée avec une introduction. Paris, 1887.

Vie d'Antoine Watteau. Publiée pour la première fois d'après le manuscrit autographe de M. de Caylus. Paris, 1887.

Lettres inédites d'Euler à d'Alembert. Publiées avec notice. Rome-Paris, 1887.

La verité sur le Marquis de Sade. Paris, 1887.

Lettres inédites de Lagrange. Paris, 1887.

Lettres inédites de Laplace. Avec notice sur les manuscrits de Pingré. Paris, 1887.

185

Bibliography

Les Voyages de Balthasar de Monconys. Documents pour l'histoire de la science, avec une introduction. Paris, 1887.

"Deux pages inédites de la vie de Frédéric le Grand." Cited by J.-F. Revel, *L'Oeil,* 1964, but which we were unable to confirm.

1888   "Lettre à Monsieur le Prince D. Balthasar Boncompagni sur divers points d'histoire des mathématiques." Place of publication unknown; advertised in inside back cover of *Cercle chromatique.*

"Rapporteur esthétique et sensation de forme." *La revue indépendânte* (April, 1888), pp. 73–90.

"Cercle chromatique et sensation de couleur." *La revue indépendante* (May, 1888), pp. 238–89.

"Harmonie de couleurs." *La revue indépendante* (June, 1888), pp. 458–78.

Cercle chromatique présentant tous les compléments et toutes les harmonies de couleurs avec une introduction sur la théorie générale du contraste, du rythme et de la mesure. Paris: Ch. Verdin, 1888. Also in large folio edition without the lengthy avant-propos.

Rapporteur esthétique, permettant l'étude et la rectification de toutes formes avec une introduction sur les applications à l'art industriel, à l'histoire de l'art, à l'interprétation de la méthode graphique. Paris: G. Seguin, 1888.

1889   "Sur la dynamogenie et l'inhibition." *Comptes rendus de l'Academie des Sciences* 108 (January 7, 1889):70–71.

"Sur un cercle chromatique, un rapporteur et un triple décimètre esthétiques." *Comptes rendus de l'Academie des Sciences* 108 (January 28, 1889):169–71.

Échelles dynamométriques, permettant de doser rigoureusement l'état des forces des sujets avec une introduction sur la pathogénie. Paris, 1889.

"Le contraste, le rythme et la mesure." *Revue philosophique* 28 (October, 1889):356–81.

1890   "Esthétique et psychophysique." *Revue philosophique* 29 (1890):332–36.

"Société de psychologie physiologique: sur une loi générale des réactions psycho-motrice." *Revue philosophique* 30 (1890):107–11.

Sur une loi générale des réactions psycho-motrice. As pre-

Bibliography

sented at the Congrès de Paris de l'Association française pour l'avancement des sciences. Paris, 1890.

*Application de nouveaux instruments de précision a l'ar-
chéologie.* Paris, 1890.

1891   *Harmonie de formes et de couleurs.* Démonstrations pra-
tiques avec le rapporteur esthétique et le cercle chromatique. Paris, 1891.

*Instruction sur les harmonies de lumière, de couleur, et de
forme.* Publiée sous les auspices du Ministre du commerce, de l'industrie et des colonies, en vue de l'introduction de ces études dans l'enseignement technique.
Listed as "in preparation," with plates by P. Signac, back
inside cover of the preceding, *Harmonie de formes.* . . .
Probably the same as the work cited by Herbert, *Neo-
Impression,* p. 140, entitled *L'education du sens des
formes,* on which Signac collaborated with Henry and
which was published in 1891, though the Louvre *Signac*
catalogue (1933) does not list such a work in its list of
"Travaux en collaboration avec Charles Henry."

"Réponse à l'enquête de Jules Huret sur l'évolution de la
littérature francaise." *L'écho de Paris.* June, 1891. Reprinted in *L'Art moderne* (25 October, 1891).

1891–1922 *Oeuvres de Fermat.* Publiées par les soins de MM. Paul
Tannery et Charles Henry sous les auspices du Ministre
de l'Instruction publique. Vol. 1 (1891), Vol. 2 (1894),
Vol. 3 (1896), Vol. 4 (1912), Supplement (1922).

1893   "Le Problème et les méthodes générales d'une psychologie
physiologique." *Revue scientifique* (February, 1893).

1894   "À travers les sciences et l'industrie: *Systèmes nerveux et
maladies,* du Manuel Leven." *La revue blanche* 6
(1894):160–67.

"À travers les sciences et l'industrie: un procédé pratique
du filigranage applicable aux éditions de luxe—parfums
artificiels—pourquoi *Au-dessus des forces humains* est
un drame profond." *La Revue blanche* 6 (1894):254–58.

"À travers les sciences et l'industrie: La Voix modifiée par
les inhalations, du Dr. A. Sandras." *La Revue blanche*
6 (1894):362–67.

1894–95 "Quelque details techniques à propos cyclisme." *La Revue
blanche* 6 (1894):561–67; 7:70–75, 273–78, 364–68,
459–63, 554–61; 8 (1895):235–39, 368–71.

"L'esthétique des formes." *La Revue blanche* 7 (1894):

Bibliography

118–29, 308–22, 511–25; 8 (1895):117–20. Edited in 1895 under the title *Quelques aperçus sur l'esthétique des formes,* with drawings and calculations by Paul Signac.

Abrégé de la théorie des fonctions elliptiques à l'usage des candidats à la licence ès sciences mathématiques. Paris, 1895.

"À travers les sciences et l'industrie: La Fatigue intellectuelle et physique, d'après M. Mosso." *La revue blanche* 7 (1894):171–77.

"L'Oeuvre ophtalmologique de Thomas Young." *La revue blanche* 8 (1895):473–77.

1897 *Les Rayons Röntgens.* Paris, 1897.

1906 *Mesure des capacités intellectuelles et énergétiques.* . . . Brussels: Institut Solvay, 1906.

1908 *La loi de petits nombres. Recherches sur le sens de l'écart probable dans les chances simples à roulette, au trente et quarante, et en générale dans les phénomènes dépendant de causes purement accidentalles.* Brussels: Institut Solvay, 1908.

1909 *Psycho-physique et énergétique.* Paris: Institut générale psychologique, bulletin no. 1, 1909. Probably the same as *Psychobiologie et énergétique,* listed in the bibliography given at the end of "Hommage à Henry," *Cahiers de l'étoile,* as having been published in 1908.

1910 *Sensation et énergie.* Paris: Institut générale psychologique, 1910.

1911 *Mémoire et habitude.* Paris: Institut générale psychologique, 1911.

1918 *Rayonnement, gravitation, vie.* Paris: Institut gènèrale psychologique, 1918.

1920 "Le problème de la balnéothérapie." *La presse thermale et climatique.* 1920. Also reprinted in *Le courrier médical* (1920).

1921 "La lumière, la couleur, et la forme." *L'esprit nouveau* (1921), pp. 605–23, 729–36, 948–58, 1068–75. Also published as a book under the same title (1922).

1924 *Essai de généralisation de la théorie du rayonnement: résonateurs biologiques, exposition intuitive des résultats techniques essentiels de la théorie de la relativité.* Paris, 1924.

1925 "Ce que je sais de Dieu." *Cahiers contemporains* 1 (Paris, 1925).

Bibliography

1926   "Vie et survie." *Cahiers contemporains* 2 (Paris, 1926). Reprinted in *Le courrier médical.*

"Fréquences nerveuses des fonctions psychiques." *Cahiers contemporains,* 3 (Paris, 1926).

"Postface," in Robert Mirabaud, *Charles Henry et l'idéalisme scientifique.* Paris: 1926, pp. 65–78.

Selected bibliography of articles and books on Charles Henry, psychophysics, and psychophysical art and aesthetics

Excellent bibliographical material is contained in Homer, *Seurat and the Science of Painting,* and Rewald, *Post-impressionnism;* we have no intention of duplicating them, but rather look at them as basic bibliographical sources. What we list, in addition to references not cited by Rewald or Homer, are chiefly sources emphasizing the salient points in our thesis.

Articles

Aaronson, Bernard S. "Hypnotic Alterations of Space and Time." *International Journal of Parapsychology* 10 (Spring, 1968):5–36.

———. "Mysticism and Depth Perception." *Journal for the Scientific Study of Religion* 6, no. 2 (1967):246–52.

———. "Some Spatial Stereotypes of Time." Paper presented at meeting of the Eastern Psychological Association, Washington, D.C., 1968.

Argüelles, José A. "Paul Signac's *Against the Enamel of a Background Rhythmic with Beats and Angles, Tones and Colors, Portrait of M. Félix Fénéon in 1890, Opus 217.*" *Journal of Aesthetics and Art Criticism* 38, no. 1 (Fall, 1969):49–53.

Boyer, J. "Nécrologie: Charles Henry." *Revue générale des sciences pures et appliquées* 38 (January 15, 1927):1–2.

Cachin, Francoise. "The Neo-Impressionist Avant-Garde." *Art News Annual* 34 (1968):54–65.

Chipp, Herschel. "Orphism and Color Theory." *Art Bulletin* 40 (1958):55–63.

Danielou, Alain. "Influence of Sound on Consciousness." *Psychedelic Review,* no. 7 (1966):20–26.

Fénéon, Félix. "Charles Henry: notice nécrologique." *Bulletin de la vie artistique* (November 15, 1926).

Fingestein, Peter. "Spirituality, Mysticism and Non-Objective Art." *Art Journal* 21, no. 1 (Fall, 1961):1–6.

Geroult, Georges. "Du rôle des mouvements des yeux dans les émotions esthétiques." *Gazette des beaux-arts* VI 1 (1881):536ff; VI 2:82ff.

Bibliography

————. "Formes, couleurs, mouvements." *Gazette des beaux-arts* VII 1 (1882):165ff.

Hericourt, Jacques. "Projet de questionnaire psychologique." *Revue philosophique* 29 (1890):445–48.

————. "Une théorie mathématique de l'expression: le contrast, le rythme, et la mesure, d'après les travaux de M. Charles Henry." *Revue scientifique* 44 (November, 1889):586–93.

Kahn, Gustave. "Au temps du pointillisme." *Mercure de France,* April, 1924, pp. 5–22.

————. "Réponse aux symbolistes." *L'événement* (Paris), September 28, 1886.

Lachelas, Georges. Review of Charles Henry, *Cercle chromatique* and *Rapporteur esthétique. Revue philosophique* 28 (1889): 635–45.

Laforgue, Jules. "Impressionism," in Linda Nochlin, *Impressionism and Post-Impressionism, 1874–1904, Sources and Documents.* Englewood Cliffs, N. J., 1966.

Lipps, Theodore. "Sur l'espace de la perception visuelle." *Revue philosophique* 27 (1889):424ff.

Lyons, Joseph. "Paleolithic Aesthetics." *Journal of Aesthetics and Art Criticism* (Fall, 1967), pp. 107–14.

Metzner, Ralph. Review of C. Daly King, *The States of Human Consciousness. Psychedelic Review* no. 4 (1964):486–89.

Metzner, Ralph, and Leary, Timothy. "On Programming Psychedelic Experiences." *Psychedelic Review* no. 9 (1967):4–19.

Murphy, Gardner. "Human Psychology in the Context of the New Knowledge." *Main Currents in Modern Thought* 21, no. 4 (March–April, 1965):75–81.

Revel, J.-F. "Charles Henry et la science des arts." *L'Oeil* (November, 1964), pp. 20–27, 44, 58.

Sorel, Georges. "Contributions psycho-physiques à l'esthétique." *Revue philosophique* 29 (1890):561–79.

————. "Esthétique et psychophysique." *Revue philosophique* 29 (1890):182–84.

Books

Andry-Bourgeois, C. *L'oeuvre de Charles Henry et le problème de la survie.* Paris, 1931.

Babbitt, Edwin. *Principles of Light and Color.* Edited and with an introduction by Faber Birren. New Hyde Park, 1968. (First edition, 1878.)

Baudelaire, Charles. *L'Art romantique.* Paris, 1885.

Bibliography

————. *Intimate Journals*. Translated by Christopher Isherwood. Boston, 1957.

Bergson, Henri. *Matter and Memory*. New York, 1959. (First edition, Paris, 1896.)

————. *Time and Free Will, An Essay on the Immediate Data of Consciousness*. New York, 1960. (First edition, Paris, 1889.)

Berkeley, George. *Three Dialogues between Hylas and Philonous*. Chicago, 1959. (First edition, London, 1713.)

Bertholet, M. *Les origines de l'alchimie*. Paris, 1885.

Besant, Annie and Leadbeater, C. W. *Thought Forms*. London, 1901.

Blanc, Charles. *Grammaire des arts du dessin*. Paris, 1867.

Bohr, Niels. *Essays 1958/1962 on Atomic Physics and Human Knowledge*. New York, 1963.

Borges, Jorge Luis. *Other Inquisitions*. New York, 1965.

Boring, Edwin C., *The Physical Dimensions of Consciousness*. New York, 1963.

————. *Sensation and Perception in the History of Experimental Psychology*. New York, 1950.

Birren, Faber. *Color: A Survey in Words and Pictures*. New Hyde Park, 1963.

————. *Color Psychology and Color Therapy*. New Hyde Park, 1961.

Cahiers de l'étoile, "Hommage à Charles Henry," no. 13 (January–February, 1930).

Caillot, Albert. *Manuel bibliographique des sciences occultes ou psychiques*. Vol. 2. Paris, 1912.

Chaix, Marie-Antoinette. *La correspondance des arts dans la poesie contemporaine*. Paris, 1919.

Chevreul, Michel-Eugene. *De la loi du contraste simultané des couleurs et de l'assortiment des objets colorés*. Paris, 1886. (First edition, 1839.)

Collie, Michael, *Laforgue*. Glasgow, 1963.

Dampier, Sir William Cecil, *A History of Science and Its Relations with Philosophy and Religion*. Cambridge, 1966.

Delaunay, Robert. *Du cubisme à l'art abstrait*. Documents inédits publiés par Pierre Francastel. Paris, 1957.

Delboeuf, J. R. L. *Examen critique de la loi psychophysique: sa base et sa signification*. Paris, 1883.

Dufour, M. *Etude sur l'esthétique de Jules Laforgue*. Paris, 1904.

Eliade, Mircea. *Cosmos and History*. New York, 1959.

————. *Myths, Dreams and Mysteries*. New York, 1960.

————. *Yoga: Freedom and Immortality*. New York, 1959.

191

Bibliography

Evans-Wentz. *The Tibetan Book of the Great Liberation*. With psychological commentary by C. G. Jung. Oxford, 1954.

Evergreen Review 4, no. 13 (May–June, 1960), "What is 'Pataphysics?'"

Fechner, Gustav, *Elements of Psychophysics*. Translated by Helmut E. Adler, edited by Davis H. Howes and Edwin G. Boring. Vol. 1 (New York, 1966). (First edition, Leipzig, 1861.)

———. *On Life after Death*. Translated by Hugo Warnekke. Chicago, 1906. (First edition, Leipzig, 1835.)

———. *Religion of a Scientist, Selected Writings*. Edited and translated by Walter Lowrie. New York, 1946.

———. *Vorschule der Aesthetik*. Leipzig, 1876.

Fénéon, Félix. *Au-delà de l'impressionnisme*. Presentation by Françoise Cachin. Paris, 1966.

———. *Oeuvres*. Edited and with an introduction by Jean Paulhan. Paris, 1948.

Feré, C. *Sensation et Mouvement*. Paris, 1887.

Gauguin, Paul. *Intimate Journals*. London, 1923.

———. *Letters to His Wife and His Friends*. Edited by M. Malingue. New York, 1949.

Govinda, Lama Anagarika. *The Psychological Attitude of Early Buddhist Philosophy*. London, 1961.

Gregory, R. L. *Eye and Brain: the Psychology of Seeing*. New York, 1966.

Hall, G. Stanley. *Founders of Modern Psychology*. New York, 1912.

Heisenberg, *Physics and Philosophy: The Revolution in Modern Science*. New York, 1958.

Helmholtz, Hermann von. *Handbuch der Physiologischen Optik*. Leipzig, 1855–65.

———. *Popular Scientific Lectures*. New York, 1881.

Herbert, Robert L. *Neo-Impressionism*. New York, 1968.

Herrnstein, Richard J. and Boring, Edwin G. *A Source Book in the History of Psychology*. Cambridge, 1965.

Homer, William. *Seurat and the Science of Painting*. Cambridge, 1964.

Jacobi, Jolande. *The Psychology of C. G. Jung*. New Haven, 1942.

Jaensch, E. R. *Eidetic Images*. London, 1930. (First edition, 1922).

Jarry, Alfred. *Selected Works*. Edited by Roger Shattuck. New York, 1965.

Jung, C. G. *Man and His Symbols,* New York, 1964.

———. *Psychology and Alchemy*. Vol. 12 of the collected works. New York, 1953.

Jung, C. G., and Pauli, W. *The Interpretation of Nature and the*

Bibliography

Psyche: Synchronicity, an Acausal Connecting Principle (Jung), and *The Influence of Archetypal Ideas on the Scientific Theories of Kepler.* New York, 1955.

Jung, C. G., and Wilhelm, Richard. *The Secret of the Golden Flower.* New York, 1931.

Kallen, H. R. *Art and Freedom,* Vol. 2. New York, 1942.

Kahn, Gustave, *Les Dessins de Seurat.* Paris, 1928.

————. *Symbolistes et décadents.* Paris, 1902.

Kandinsky, Wassily. *On the Spiritual in Art.* New York, 1946. (First published, 1911.)

Kuhn, Thomas S. *The Structure of Scientific Revolutions.* Chicago, 1970.

Laforgue, Jules. *Lettres à un ami. 1880–1886.* Edited with an introduction and notes by G. Jean-Aubry. Paris, 1941.

————. *Oeuvres complètes.* Vols. 4, 5 (letters). Edited by G. Jean-Aubry. Paris, 1922.

Leonardo da Vinci, *Notebooks.* Edited and with commentaries by Irma A. Richter. London, 1952.

Lövgren, Sven. *The Genesis of Modernism. Seurat, Gauguin, Van Gogh and French Symbolism in the 1880's.* Uppsala, 1959.

M. Luckiesh. *Color and Its Applications.* New York, 1921.

————. *Visual Illusions. Their Causes, Characteristics and Applications.* New York, 1922.

McLuhan, Marshall. *Understanding Media.* New York, 1964.

Marey, Edouard. *Étude de la locomotion animale par la chronophotographie.* Paris, 1887.

Martin, Elizabeth P. "The Symbolist Criticism of Painting in France: 1880–95." Ph.D. dissertation, Bryn Mawr College, 1952.

Mirabaud, Robert. *Charles Henry et l'idéalisme scientifique.* Postface by Charles Henry, Appendix by Victor Delfino. Paris, 1926.

Mookerjee, Akit. *Tantra Art: Its Philosophy and Physics.* New Delhi, 1966.

Mukerjee, Radhakamal. *The Social Function of Art.* Bombay, 1948.

Musée du Louvre. *Signac.* Paris, 1963–64.

Musée Nationale de l'Art Moderne. *Kupka.* Paris, 1966.

Ostwald, Wilhelm. *Colour Science.* 2 vol. London, n.d.

Ouspensky, P. D. *In Search of the Miraculous.* New York, 1948.

————. *A New Model of the Universe: Principles of the Psychological Method in Its Application to Problems of Science, Religion and Art.* New York, 1943.

Ramsay, Warren. *Jules Laforgue and the Ironic Inheritance.* New York, 1953.

Rewald, John. *Georges Seurat.* Paris, 1948.

Bibliography

———. *Post-impressionism*. New York, 1956.

Richter, Peyton E. *Perspectives in Aesthetics, Plato to Camus*. New York, 1967.

Renchi, Vasche. *L'optique, science de la vision*. Paris, 1966.

Rood, Ogden, *Modern Chromatics*. New York, 1879. (French edition, 1881.)

Rookmaaker, *Synthetist Art Theories*. Amsterdam, 1959.

Roszak, Theodore. *The Making of a Counter-Culture*, New York, 1968.

Ruchon, François. *Jules Laforgue: sa oeuvre, sa vie*. Geneva, 1924.

Russell, John. *Seurat*. London, 1965.

Scharf, Aaron. *Creative Photography*. London, 1965.

Schmutzler, Robert. *Art nouveau*. New York, 1964.

Seuphor, Michel. *L'art abstrait*, Paris, 1948.

Signac, Paul. *De Delacroix au néo-impressionnisme*. Presentation by Françoise Cachin. Paris, 1964. (First published, 1899.)

Singer, Charles. *A Short History of Scientific Ideas to 1900*. Oxford, 1959.

Sze, Mai-Mai. *The Way of Chinese Painting*. New York, 1959.

Tucci, Giuseppe. *Theory and Practice of the Mandala, with Special Reference to the Modern Psychology of the Subconscious*. London, 1961.

Valéry, Paul. *Selected Writings*. New York, 1950.

Warrain, Francis. *L'Oeuvre psychobiophysique de Charles Henry*. Paris, 1931.

Woodroffe, Sir John (Arthur Avalon). *The Serpent Power, Being the Sat-Cakra-Nirupana and Paduka-Pancaka*. Madras, 1964. (First edition, 1918.)

Worringer, W. *Abstraction and Empathy*. London, 1953. (First published, 1908.)

———. *Form in Gothic*. New York, 1963. (First published, 1912.)

Zeller, Eduard. *Outlines of the History of Greek Philosophy*. New York, 1955. (First edition, Berlin, 1883.)

Index

Adam, Paul, 103
Aesthetics: and art history, 33; and consciousness, 127; history of, 50, 85, 87–88; problem of, 167. *See also* Art; Henry, Charles, aesthetic doctrine of; Psychophysical aesthetic
Albers, Josef, 150
Alchemy, and science, 37, 39
Apollinaire, G., 149
Arabesque. *See* Continual autogenesis, principle of
Archetypal forms, 121, 125
Archetypes, 25, 121
Aristotle, 85
Arrest, phenomena of, 168
Art: abstract, 2 n, 139, 148, 150, 152; as applied psychophysics, 33; and consciousness, 19, 33; and evolution, 129, 154; as harmonic keyboard for human body, 155; harmonic stream of, 150; and knowledge, 132; Op, 150; and science, 20, 40, 41, 73, 82; psychedelic, 150; as psychobiological projection, 145, 146, 148; psychophysical, 150. *See also* Aesthetics
Art history as historical psychology, 33
Art nouveau, 131, 144–45, 146, 150;
as dynamogenous style, 129–30; and psychophysics, 28
Astrology and science, 37, 38

Babbitt, E., 64
Barbevara, 103
Baudelaire, Charles, 9, 60, 87, 88; "Correspondances," 99
Bergson, Henri, 145; *Essai sur les données immédiates de la conscience,* 21–22; and psychophysics, 22
Berkeley, Lord, 57 n
Bernard, Claude, 5, 32, 56, 65
Bert, Paul, 5, 100
Bicycle. *See* Cycles, theory of
Biological romanticism, 145
Blake, William, 166 n. *See also* Newton, Sir Isaac
Blanc, Charles, 2 n, 87
Blavatsky, Madame, 151
Bohr, Neils, 39; and law of complementarity, 16
Borges, Jorge Luis, 42, 140
Bossuet, 35, 37
Brown, Sequard, M., 167
Buddha, 8, 56
Buddhism, 59; and psychophysics, 11, 15 n, 62–63

Carroll, Lewis, 24

Index

Cartesian system. *See* Science, history of

Casanova, Jacques, 41; family of, 47 n

Caylus, Comte de, and rediscovery of encaustic technique, 47–48

Chakras, 140

Charcot, J. M., 103

Chardin, J. B. S., 47

Chevreul, M. E., 94, 95, 116, 117, 164

Christophe, Jules, 103

Circle: as biopsychic norm, 139, 140, 141; functions of, 91, 92, 109 n, 119, 128, 137–38, 140, 147, 148; history of, 139. *See also* Cycles, theory of; Mandala

Clerk-Maxwell, J., 63–64

Club des hydropaths, 5

Cochin, C. N., 40, 77

Consciousness: alteration of, 18–19; evolution of, 26; history of, 100; nature of, 144; psychology of, 142 n; states of, 12, 18, 30 n, 161. *See also* Henry, Charles, definition of consciousness, theory of consciousness

Continual autogenesis, principle of, 97, 131, 133, 135

Correspondences, theory of, 100

Cros, Charles, 42, 60

Cubism, 146

Cycles, theory of, 4 n, 42, 91–92, 106 n, 110, 111, 119, 128, 137, 138, 144, 148, 172. *See also* Circle

d'Alembert, 69

Dampier, W. C., 34

Dante, 139, 144, 178

Darwin, Charles, 9, 15, 71, 85

Debussy, Claude, 91

Degas, Edgar, 23, 60

Delaunay, Robert, 118; early development of, 147; "On Light," 146–47, 149

Delbouef, Jean, 21

Descartes, René, 10, 16, 18, 34, 35, 48, 82, 83, 172; theorem on co-ordinates, 46. *See also* Cartesian system

Diderot, aesthetic of, 47

Disney, Walt, *Fantasia*, 154

Dorra, Henri, 2–3

Dubois-Pillet, Albert, 103

Duchamp (brothers), 149

Dujardin, Edouard, 103

Dynamogeny, 89, 92, 112. *See also* Henry, Charles, theory of dynamogeny and inhibition

Edison, T. A., 64

Eidetic images, 28 n, 150

Energy: and perception, 137; theories of, 170–71

Ephrussi, Charles, 70

Evolution, law of, 173. *See also* Henry, Charles, law of evolution, and theory of evolution

Faustroll, Dr., 24, 30

Fechner, Gustav Theodor, 11 n, 15, 22, 25, 29, 35, 63, 70 n, 83, 85, 88, 102, 113, 140, 142 n

———, works by: *Elements of psychophysics*, 15, 20; *Vorschule der Aesthetik*, 29 n; *Zend Avesta*, 15 n, 25 n. *See also* Psychophysics, definition of

Fénéon, Félix, 5, 74, 81, 82, 98, 100, 103, 125 n, 132, 133, 134; on Charles Henry, 23

Feré, Charles, 168

Ferté, M., 80

Forain, Jules, 60

Fourier, Charles, 129 n

Fragonard, J. H., portraits of, 47

Galileo, 40

Gauguin, Paul, 80, 90, 129; and "papier de Gauguin," 79

Geroult, Georges, 61 n, 88, 115 n

Gesamtkunstwerk, 52, 90, 96, 154

Ghil, René, 91, 100, 125 n, 179

Gleizes, A., 149

196

Index

Goethe, J. W. von, 102, 117
Golden section, 93, 112
Govinda, Lama, 8 n, 29 n, 56
Greenaway, Kate, 60
Greuze, J. B., 47
Gurdjieff, 142 n

Hanslick, E., 88, 97
Hartmann, E. von, 59, 63, 71, 100, 102, 117
Hallucinations, 127
Heisenberg, Werner, 16 n
Helmholtz, H. von, 20, 28, 63, 71, 89, 94, 99, 117, 119, 125; theory of musical vibrations, 98
Henry, Charles: aesthetic doctrine of, 1–3, 7, 10, 23–24, 27–28, 41, 45–46, 51–52, 69–70, 74–75, 76, 82–85, 89–90, 92, 94, 96–97, 99, 101, 107, 110–12, 114, 120–22, 126–27, 129, 132, 139, 145, 151; and alchemy, 35 n, 37; analysis of auditory experience, 122, 123–25; analysis of visual sensation, 115–19; on art and social change, 153–54; on art as therapy, 154–56, 181; and art of symbolist era, 90–91, 96, 99, 100, 103, 104, 178–79; on beauty, 157; and Bergson, 22, 26; and biology, 101–2; and Buddhism, 8, 62; color theory of, 94–95, 116, 118, 135–36; and Cros, 47 n; definition of aesthetic doctrine, 51; definition of art and science, 84; definition of consciousness, 109, 156; defintion of continuity and discontinuity, 172; definition of dynamogeny and inhibition, 167–68; definition of rhythm, 23; definition of rhythm and measure, 174; description of evolutionary process, 128–29; and doctrine of harmony, 143, 148; and doctrine if psychomagnetic reactions, 90 n; and dualism, 83, 101; early friendship with Laforgue, 54–55, 56, 58, 59, 60, 61, 64, 67, 69–70, 76–77; and eighteenth-century culture, 46–47, 48, 68; erudite publications, 40–42; and formulation of aesthetic problem, 88, 105; on future of art, 177–78; and Gauguin, 80–81; general method and research of, 33, 43; historical studies of, 93; and history of art, 40; and history of mathematics, 8, 33–34, 36; and history of science, 26, 32, 33, 35–36, 48; influence of aesthetic doctrine, 118, 130; influence on modern art, 146, 148–49, 150; on language, 180–81; law of evolution of, 128; lectures on aesthetics, 78, 80, 81; as librarian of Sorbonne, 41–42; mathematical publications of, 41; mathematical theory of, 45; on moral/aesthetic imperative, 114, 115, 119; on music, 98; musical studies of, 51; and mysticism, 27; and neo-impressionism, 2, 82, 97, 98; and neopythagoreanism, 9, 91; and 'Pataphysics, 30–32; on poetry and mathematics, 23–24; and psychophysics, 17, 21, 22, 24, 29, 39; and psychotherapy, 25; and Pythagoras, 44, 85; and scientific method, 16, 33, 35; scientific research of, 5–6, 60 n, 64; social implications of aesthetic doctrine of, 49–50; on social function of art, 180; theory of consciousness, 142; and theory of continuity and discontinuity, 112–13, 114, 116, 125–28, 136, 137, 167; theory of contrast, 108–9, 114, 116, 127, 173; and theory of directions, 88–89, 90, 91, 93, 101, 106, 107, 108, 115, 118, 121; and theory of dynamogeny and inhibition, 107, 110–11, 114, 118, 125–28, 134, 144, 146; and theory of evolution, 9, 10, 11, 26; and theory of interior work, 105–6;

197

Index

Index

Marey, E., 106, 109, 111, 168 n
Matter, definition of, 173–74
Metzinger, J., 149
Michelangelo, 85
Monet, Claude, 60, 70 n; and psychophysics, 20
Moreas, Jean, 103, 125 n
Morris, William, 129
Mullezer, Mme. See Multzer, Mme
Multzer, Mme, 5, 58, 61, 77
Murphy, Gardner, 13, 14
Mystical experience, psychophysiological description of, 123, 155–56
Mysticism: definition of, 24–25; and materialism, 25

Neo-impressionism, 28, 75, 79, 90, 93, 117, 132, 139; and technique of color photography, 47 n
Newton, Sir Isaac, 32, 33, 34; and William Blake, 34 n

Octave, theory of, 138
Op art. See Art, Op
Optical illusions, 165–66. See also Eidetic images; Hallucinations; Perception, cycles of
Orphism, 146, 149
Ouspensky, P. D., 1 n, 138 n

Painting, abstract. See Art, abstract
Parmenides, 140
Pascal, 35, 139
'Pataphysics, 23 n, 30; definition of, 31
Pauli, Wolfgang, 38, 39
Perception, cycles of, 136–37
Perception and motion, 166
Physics and non-Western modes of consciousness, 18
Picabia, F., 149
Pissarro, Camille, 78, 138
Planck, Max, 39; quantum theory of, 45
Plato, 85, 139
Plotinus, 15 n, 147
Poe, E. A., 87, 88

Portrait of Fénéon. See Signac, Paul, Portrait of Fénéon
Pre-Socratics, 139
Psychedelics and psychophysics, 141 n
Psychic functions, continuity and discontinuity of, 163–64
Psychology: development of, 13–14, 15 n; of the unconscious, 25
Psychomathematics, 8
Psychomotor reactions, law of, 18, 114, 144
Psychone, 92
Psychophysical aesthetic, 28, 29, 71, 144–45, 161; basic assumptions of, 76, 106; definition of, 45–46; elements of, 169; and global art, 157; social implications of, 161; in treatment of social problems, 152–53. See also Henry, Charles, aesthetic doctrine of; Psychophysics
Psychophysics: and behaviorism, 14, 28 n; and Buddhism, 8 n, 11, 15 n, 29 n; definition of, 10–11, 12, 15, 17, 22, 28–29, 46; and doctrine of harmony, 84–85, 86, 143; and history of culture, 39; and literature, 125 n; and nineteenth-century culture, 3, 12, 17, 20, 21; and Oriental thought, 11 n, 15 n; outer and inner, 17. See also Consciousness; Fechner, Gustav; Henry, Charles
Ptolemy, 125
Pythagoras, 8, 9, 10, 36 n, 44, 56, 85, 125, 172

Quantum mechanics, 17

Rameau, 85; musical theories of, 48 n, 51
Raymond, Maurice, 103
Rewald, John, 2, 175
Rimbaud, Arthur, 179; "Vowels," 100
Roberval, 37
Rood, Ogden, 94

199

Index

between biology and physics, painting and music, sensation and action." To the Parisian symbolists of the 1880s, he was the synthesizing genius who provided both the theorems and the proofs of that symbolic calculus which would lead to the apprehension of beauty through the sensory interfusion described as synesthesia.

Mr. Argüelles's work represents the first historical consideration of the phenomenon of psychophysics and its place in the history of Western thought and aesthetics. The study includes a portion of Henry's central work on psychophysics, *Le cercle chromatique*, a revealing interview with Henry by Jules Huret titled "Inquiry Concerning the Future of Literature," and a bibliography of the works of Charles Henry.

JOSÉ A. ARGÜELLES was awarded his Ph.D. in art history at the University of Chicago in 1969. He is now coordinator of the Man and Art Program at the Evergreen State College in Washington. He has worked with his wife, Miriam, as a painter and illustrator, and their work has been exhibited in several museums and galleries. They have also written and published a book, *Mandala*.

ISBN: 0-226-02757-0
Printed in U.S.A.

Paul Signac's *Against the Enamel of a Background Rhythmic with Beats and Angles, Tones and Colors. Portrait of M. Félix Fénéon in 1890, Opus 217.*
Private collection, New York
Photograph by Charles Uht